HOMEOPATHY
FOR
BACK AND
NECK PAIN

BOOK YOUR PLACE ON OUR WEBSITE
AND MAKE THE
READING CONNECTION!

We've created a customized website just for our very special readers, where you can get the inside scoop on everything that's going on with Zebra, Pinnacle and Kensington books.

When you come online, you'll have the exciting opportunity to:

- View covers of upcoming books
- Read sample chapters
- Learn about our future publishing schedule (listed by publication month *and author*)
- Find out when your favorite authors will be visiting a city near you
- Search for and order backlist books from our online catalog
- Check out author bios and background information
- Send e-mail to your favorite authors
- Meet the Kensington staff online
- Join us in weekly chats with authors, readers and other guests
- Get writing guidelines
- AND MUCH MORE!

**Visit our website at
http://www.kensingtonbooks.com**

HOMEOPATHY FOR BACK AND NECK PAIN

Ursula Stone

Kensington Books
Kensington Publishing Corp.
http://www.kensingtonbooks.com

KENSINGTON BOOKS are published by

Kensington Publishing Corp.
850 Third Avenue
New York, NY 10022

Kensington and the K logo Reg. U.S. Pat. & TM Off.

First Printing: August, 1999
10 9 8 7 6 5 4 3 2 1

Printed in the United States of America

DISCLAIMER

This book is intended as a source of information. Every effort has been made to include the most up-to-date and accurate information; however, it is impossible to include everything in a basic guide, and there can be no guarantee that this information won't change in time as a result of ongoing medical research.

All matters regarding your health require medical supervision. The information presented herein is intended to supplement, not replace, the medical advice of trained professionals. Before you adopt any of the ideas, procedures, or suggestions contained in this book, consult your own physician to make sure that they are appropriate for you.

Any adoption of the information herein is at the reader's discretion. Neither the author nor the publisher assume any responsibility or liability arising directly or indirectly from the use of the information in this book.

The highest ideal of cure is rapid, gentle and permanent restoration of the health, or removal and annihilation of the disease in its whole extent, in the shortest, most reliable, and most harmless way, on easily comprehensible principles.

—Dr. Samuel Hahnemann

Homeopathy is one of the rare medical approaches which carries no penalties—only benefits.

—Yehudi Menuhin, violinist and
Past President of the
Hahnemann Society, U.K.

Homeopathy cures a greater number of cases than any other method of treatment.

—Mahatma Gandhi

You may honestly feel grateful that homeopathy has survived the attempts of the allopathists (orthodox physicians) to destroy it.

—Mark Twain

To like things like, whatever one may ail; there is certain help.

—Johann Wolfgang von Goethe, *Faust*

Through the like, disease is produced, and through the application of the like it is cured.

—Hippocrates

Contents

PART THREE: THE MATERIA MEDICA, A CATALOG OF REMEDIES

Part Four: Additional Information

INTRODUCTION

Homeopathy was introduced in the United States in the 1820s by a German doctor, Constantine Hering. In 1844, the first national medical association in the United States, the American Institute of Homeopathy, was founded. By the turn of the twentieth century, almost one quarter of all doctors were practicing homeopathy, and there were 22 homeopathic schools throughout the country in cities such as Chicago, Philadelphia, and Ann Arbor.

The discovery and widespread use of antibiotics eclipsed homeopathy, and by the 1920s its practice was largely abandoned in America. (It continued to flourish in Europe, however, especially in England.) The remedies were given legal status in 1938, and their manufacture and distribution is still governed by the FDA. So although there are no accredited training programs solely in homeopathy in the United States, anyone who is trained and licensed as a health care practitioner and has authority to prescribe medicines can prescribe homeopathic remedies as part of his medical practice. Certification programs, some of which are quite rigorous, are not accredited. People who learn homeopathy through these programs but are not licensed health care practitioners can be helpful as consultants. They can assist you or your doctor in identifying useful remedies. Homeopathy can be a beneficial adjunct to conventional medicine—remedies can be used to alleviate the side effects of chemotherapy or radiation treatment, to help the body clear anesthesia after surgery, or to help bones heal after a fracture.

If you decide to try homeopathy, you should limit it to self-care for non-life-threatening, acute illnesses— colds, headaches, or upset stomachs, for example—and injuries such as sprains, bruises, and cuts that don't require stitches. Severe or chronic illnesses and injuries should always be evaluated and monitored by a doctor.

Homeopathy is an art as much as it is a science. It is important to work with someone who is experienced as well as trained in the practice, someone whom you trust, and with whom you can be absolutely frank about the totality of your health. The Resources section in the back of this book lists a variety of organizations that can provide you with more information or help you locate a reputable practitioner.

PART ONE

HOMEOPATHY

FREQUENTLY ASKED QUESTIONS

What is homeopathy?

Homeopathy is a medical system that treats illness and injury with specially prepared substances called remedies. The root words *homeo* and *pathy* mean "similar suffering" and reflect the foremost idea in the treatment philosophy, usually stated as "like cures like." The guiding principles of homeopathy—like cures like, minimal doses, single medicines, and prescribing based on an assessment of the totality of symptoms—were established by its founder Dr. Samuel Hahnemann and form an effective, cohesive philosophy that has remained unchanged for more than 100 years.

The remedies, most of which are derived from plants, can be used to treat or to augment treatment for the full range of human ailments from a simple cold or sprained ankle to terminal illnesses and mental health.

As with any medical system, however, some conditions can be treated safely at home, while others are best left to the care of trained and experienced professionals. Persistent, severe, or recurring conditions should be evaluated and treated by your physician and, if you choose to augment that treatment, by an experienced homeopath. Before undertaking any medical therapy, discuss it with your doctor and your homeopath. And once the treatment is under way, keep both of them informed about any reactions that result.

How did homeopathy get started?

Samuel Hahnemann (1755–1843), a German doctor and chemist, founded homeopathy. He defined its philosophy and procedures in a book called *Organon of Medicine*. ("Organon" is a term used in philosophy for a set of logical requirements for scientific demonstration, or a body of principles of scientific or philosophic investigation.) Hahnemann began the research and experiments that homeopathy is based on in 1790, and he continued to refine the principles and practice of homeopathy throughout his long life. He revised his *Organon of Medicine* for the sixth and last time before his death at age 83.

Dr. Hahnemann enjoyed an early and successful career practicing the standard medicine of his day, even serving as personal physician to some of Germany's royal court. Nevertheless, he saw that the medicine he practiced— bloodletting and cathartic dosing with mercury, arsenic, sulfur, belladonna, and other toxic chemicals—often did more harm than good. Disenchanted with medicine, he retired from practice. To support his family, he turned a gift for languages into a successful career as a translator of medical and scientific material.

While translating a work by a noted physiologist, he was startled by the doctor's assertion that Peruvian bark (cinchona, a source of quinine) was effective against malaria because it was bitter and astringent. Ever the scientist, Hahnemann made a concoction that was even more bitter and astringent than Peruvian bark, then demonstrated that it was useless against malaria. The curative property, he now knew, lay elsewhere. Intrigued, he began taking small quantities of Peruvian bark and soon began to suffer with a persistent headache and cyclic chills, fever, and sweats—the classic symptoms of malaria. This physiological reaction sparked an intuitive leap: Hahnemann wondered if there might be a connection between the bark's ability to provoke a healthy body into counterfeiting malaria and its efficacy in curing it.

He gathered a group of people willing to help him test his idea and began a series of provings (what are now called clinical trials) in which he and they ingested small quantities of various "medicines" and kept meticulous records about their physical condition. When Dr. Hahnemann gathered these records together and analyzed them, he found that when healthy people take particular medicines, they generate symptoms that mirror the illness for which the medicine is used. Belladonna, for example, used to treat fever and conjunctivitis, caused fevers and inflamed eyes. When the subjects stopped taking the test medicine, their symptoms disappeared.

Having seen "symptoms" in healthy people, Dr. Hahnemann began thinking that these characteristic reactions were separate from disease, that symptoms were what the body did to combat illness, not the illness itself. This idea led to the primary tenet of homeopathy, what Hahnemann called the law of similars and what is popularly stated as "like cures like."

What is the law of similars?

Stated simply, the law maintains that a substance which causes an illness when taken in overdose by a healthy person, can stimulate the body to self-cure if it is taken in small doses by someone who is ill. Though controversial, this idea was not new in the eighteenth century. Hippocrates, the fourth-century physician revered as the "Father of Medicine" said, "Through the like, disease is produced, and through the application of the like it is cured." Paracelsus, a fifteenth-century Swiss physician, wrote: "bring together the same anatomy of the herbs and the same anatomy of the illness into one order. This simile gives you an understanding of the way in which you shall heal." Folk medicine holds that you treat a fever with heat—the medical application of the Native American sweat lodge. And twentieth-century medicine applies the principle under certain conditions: Allergy sufferers are given injections of the things they are allergic to; vaccinations introduce viruses so that the body can create antibodies to fight them; gold, which can cause joint pain, is used to relieve arthritis.

Hahnemann's contribution to this concept was his perception that symptoms are not the disease itself. As part of the disease process, symptoms represent the body's best efforts to combat the disease—what we now call the immune response—and any medicines that are used should be chosen for their power to assist the body's efforts. For example, mucus is one way that the body traps and expels pathogens (disease-causing microbes). When treating a cold or an allergy, a homeopath will suggest a remedy that enhances and accelerates mucus production, not a decongestant to abort it.

How is homeopathy different from regular medicine?

Homeopathy and standard medicine, sometimes called allopathy, do not diverge point-by-point, but in the philosophy as a whole. Any treatment from a classic homeopath will conform with all four of the main homeopathic principles—like cures like, minimal doses, single medicines prepared according to homeopathic practice, and prescribing based on an assessment of the totality of symptoms. Treatments from allopathic doctors may conform with some, but not with others. For example, virtually all doctors agree that vaccinations are useful in preventing the relevant viral infection, an example of like curing like. But this treatment cannot be considered homeopathic because the vaccines are not prepared in accordance with homeopathic pharmaceutics, the vaccines may be mixed (as with DPT, the diptheria-pertussis-tetanus vaccine), and the vaccines are administered prophylactically, in the absence of symptoms. Other points of difference arise from the preparation of homeopathic remedies and from the standards for dosages.

How are the remedies made?

Homeopathic medicines are primarily derived from plants, but some are made from minerals, such as calcium, gold, iron, and various salts, or from certain animal products, such as bee or snake venom. There are more than 2,000 remedies derived from various sources.

Dr. Hahnemann wanted to find the smallest effective doses of his medicines. He adamantly believed this would allow for the greatest benefit with the least harm. Through carefully monitored experiments, he evolved a systematic practice of diluting and succussing (a form of agitating) the materials of the remedies that reduced harmful effects while increasing their potency. In homeopathy, this process of alternately diluting and succussing the solution is called *potentizing*.

When working with plants, Dr. Hahnemann began by

making a mother tincture: He steeped the plant material in water or alcohol to produce a concentrated solution. Then he diluted the tincture in specific ratios. When working with insoluble materials such as minerals, the substance is mixed with a milk sugar base and ground, or triturated, with a mortar and pestle. The various potencies are achieved by timing the grinding, placing the resulting paste in solution to make a tincture, then diluting it according to the established ratios. These ratios persist today in the X-scale, C-scale, and M-scale remedy potencies. ("X" stands for 10, "C" for 100, and "M" for 1000.)

In the X-scale, 1 drop of the mother tincture was diluted in 9 drops of pure water to make a 1X solution. Then one drop was taken from the 1X and added to 9 drops of pure water to make a 2X solution. One drop of 2X was added to 9 drops of water to make 3X, and so on. This process was repeated to create a range of strengths for the medicines. The same process is used to make C-scale and M-scale remedies, except in the C-scale the dilution ratio is 1 drop to 99 drops, and in the M-scale, it is 1 to 999.

The second part of the process seems a little mystical and is the source of much of the controversy surrounding homeopathy. Dilution was not sufficient to create effective remedies, extreme dilution, in fact, destroys the substance. Additional experimentation revealed that agitating the solution by tapping the bottom of the vial against a moderately hard surface (such as a book) allowed the medicine to retain efficacy despite extreme dilution. This tapping is called "succussion," from a Latin word that means "to shake from beneath." Hahnemann discovered that the more he diluted and succussed, the stronger the remedy became; and he developed protocols for the number of succussions that should follow each dilution.

READING THE LABEL

The manufacture and distribution of homeopathic remedies is overseen by the Federal Drug Administration (FDA) and the Homeopathic Pharmacopoeia of the United States (HPUS).

Remedy labels include the name of the remedy, the potency (X-, C-, or M-scale), a lot number, directions for use, and some commonsense warnings, such as "Keep Out of the Reach of Children."

The FDA requires an expiration date, which will be stamped on the vial. Homeopathic remedies are reputed to stay potent for decades, however. If you want to use a remedy that has been stored for a long time, shake the vial before taking the remedy. This informal succussion will restore the potency.

Under "Indications" will be a list of up to three conditions for which the remedy can be used. Since there simply isn't room on the vial to provide full details about the remedy picture, consult the *Materia Medica* later in this book or one of the classic texts (*see:* Bibliography) for complete information about the individual remedies.

Why does succussion increase the strength of the remedy?

In the *Organon of Medicine*, Hahnemann discussed the presence of the "vital force," the spark that distinguishes animate from inanimate matter. Someone in possession of the vital force is alive; absent the vital force, one is dead. Health is the vital force serenely at work; illness is the vital force "deranged by . . . an agent inimical to life." It is this force, this energy, that Hahnemann believed is separated from the material substance by dilution, animated by succussion, and imprinted on the medium used for the remedy (usually milk sugar).

The vital force present in each substance has a unique pattern, and the pattern has a distinct curative property. Hahnemann compared it with magnetism:

> The medicinal property of those material substances which we call medicines proper, relates only to their energy to call out alteration in the well-being of animal life. . . . Just as the nearness of a magnetic pole can communicate only magnetic energy to the steel (namely, by a kind of infection) but cannot communicate other properties (for instance, more hardness or ductility, etc.). And thus every special medicinal substance alters through a kind of infection, that well-being of man in a peculiar manner exclusively its own and not in a manner peculiar to another medicine, as certainly as the nearness of the child ill with small-pox will communicate to a healthy child only small-pox and not measles.

Contemporary practitioners make an analogy with sympathetic vibration: The string of an instrument keyed to a particular note will vibrate in the presence of that sound, even if it is not the source of that sound. So too will the vital force of one organism resonate with the analogous vital force of another to restore health. This vibration pattern is embedded in the remedy through the prescribed combination of dilution and succussion.

Which potencies are the strongest?

The homeopathic principle is that the more you dilute and succuss, the stronger the medicine becomes; therefore, the M-scale is the strongest, and the X-scale is the mildest.

Within each scale, higher numbers indicate more dilutions; so, 12X is stronger than 6X, 200C is stronger than 30C, and 2M is stronger than 1M.

How do I know which potency to use?

Another of the guiding principles of homeopathy is minimal dosing, that is, you should take the lowest possible dose the fewest number of times to restore your health. Hahnemann called this the "law of infinitesimals" and observed that high potencies, even of correctly chosen remedies, can "prove injurious by its mere magnitude." He declined to give specific guidelines for dosages beyond recommending seeking the minutest amount and said that: "It is impossible . . . to tabulate in advance all imaginable cases. Pure experiment, careful observation of the sensitiveness of each patient and accurate experience can alone determine this *in each individual case*." In other words, you are the best judge of how the remedy and your illness are interacting.

Some general guidelines have evolved over the decades that homeopathy has been in use. Use the following suggestions, beginning treatment with the lowest potency. As you become familiar with the remedies and the effects of different potencies, you will be better able to make effective selections. If necessary, the remedies can be taken more frequently to sustain their effects. X- and C-scale potencies are commonly available at health food stores and some pharmacies. M-scale remedies are used to address chronic conditions or entrenched, long-standing illnesses (whether mental or physical). Because their effects are so profound, M-scale remedies are not commonly available over the counter. They should be taken only under the supervision of an experienced homeopath.

The X-scale and lower potencies of the C-scale (12C) are helpful with people who are greatly debilitated or who are fragile even when they are healthy—young children and the elderly, for example. They are also helpful with illnesses and injuries such as skin rashes or muscle sprains that are considered external or superficial in homeopathic terms (*see*: Planes of Illness). The X-scale and the midrange of the C-scale (30C) are appropriate for normally robust people with acute illnesses.

The higher ranges of the C-scale (200C and above) can be used in cases where there is a broad overlap between your symptoms and the remedy picture or when acute symptoms are severe or incapacitating: high fever, frequent vomiting, intractable nasal mucus, pounding headache, for example.

What is a "remedy picture"?

In the course of proving a remedy, a variety of symptoms are elicited and cataloged. They are organized in the Materia Medica by the part of the body affected: mind, head, eyes, ears, nose, face, mouth, stomach, abdomen, stool, male/female, respiratory, heart, back, extremities, and skin. An additional category—called "Modalities"—addresses the things that make you feel better or worse, which may include eating or not eating, food cravings or aversions, weather conditions, sleep patterns, time of day or night.

This catalog of symptoms is the remedy picture. When selecting a remedy, you or your homeopath will review these descriptions, looking for the one that best matches the totality of your symptoms.

PLANES OF ILLNESS

Illnesses can afflict any level of your being. Contemporary homeopaths use the following scale, published by George Vithoulkas in 1980, to assess the severity of an illness. The mental plane is the deepest level; the physical plane is the most superficial. There are degrees of depth within each plane as well. Knowing how deep the problem is helps you determine the potency of remedy. In general, the deeper the problem, the higher the potency of the appropriate remedy. Within each column, the conditions are listed in order from the deepest to the most superficial.

Physical	Emotional	Mental
Brain	Suicidal depression	Confusion
Heart	Apathy	Delirium
Endocrine	Sadness	Paranoia
Liver	Anguish	Delusions
Lungs	Phobias	Lethargy
Kidneys	Anxiety	Dullness
Bone	Irritability	Lack of
Muscle	Dissatisfaction	Concentration
Skin		Forgetfulness
		Absentmindedness

What is meant by "totality of symptoms"?

"Totality of symptoms" is the fourth basic precept of homeopathy. When you become unwell, you develop a set of symptoms that reflect your body's efforts to restore its innate state of health. The symptoms are specific to the illness—a cold and a flu, for example, are similar but distinct—but they are also specific to you, to the particular way that you manifest the illness. Homeopathy has always been a holistic system and takes all differences into account. Attention is given to the way an illness disrupts your mental and emotional health as well as your physical condition. For example, if you go to an allopathic doctor with a sore throat, you might not think to mention that your hands itch. This point would be relevant to a homeopath and could be the difference between a remedy that helps and one that doesn't. While taking your case, a homeopath will ask questions designed to discover a broad range of symptoms. In self-care of acute illnesses, you would use the same process, just remember to choose remedies according to the immediate symptom picture, even in an ongoing illness.

Physical symptoms let you know whether you have a cold or the flu, a headache or a sinus infection, a pulled muscle or a broken bone. Other symptoms reveal your mental and emotional states—you want to be left alone or you want someone to bring you drinks and read you stories until you feel better. You may feel anxious or depressed, or perhaps normally you are quick-witted, but a cold makes you dull and forgetful.

When you are sick you might seek particular environments because they help you feel better: You sit by an open window or turn on a fan because the moving air is soothing. Or you bundle up in blankets and lie still in the dark because that is soothing. You will also avoid things that make you feel worse; for example, you may be very hungry but refuse to eat because you can't keep anything down.

The weather or the time of day may influence how you feel. You might feel better in cool damp weather, worse in dry weather, and terrible if it's windy, no matter what the temperature or humidity. You may feel worse in the morning and better as the day goes on or just the opposite.

You may also manifest symptoms that seem contradictory; for example, you may have chills but crave cold drinks, or you may have a frequent, urgent desire to urinate, but urinating is painful and scanty. In homeopathy, these unexpected combinations are called peculiars and are often the most significant factors for determining an appropriate remedy.

The remedy pictures include a broad array of physical, mental, and emotional effects. Compare the array of symptoms you are experiencing to the effects described in the remedy profiles in the Materia Medica (Part Three). The remedy with greatest overlap with your condition is the one that will be the most help in relieving your illness.

Is a compound remedy more effective than a single remedy?

Dr. Hahnemann was opposed to using compound medicines. In the *Organon* he says: "In no case under treatment is it necessary and *therefore not permissible* to administer to a patient more than *one single simple medicinal* substance at a time."

In accordance with this principle, classic homeopaths always look for the one remedy best suited to a particular case and, as has been demonstrated, because each remedy influences a broad range of symptoms, a single well-chosen remedy will be effective over the range of those symptoms.

However, compound remedies can be helpful to the layman if you are having trouble identifying a remedy or in deciding between two or more. A compound medicine will broaden your chances of stumbling on one that works, but it may also result in so-called side effects—an inadvertent proving of the unnecessary medication.

How does a homeopath decide which remedy will be the most helpful?

Your homeopath will ask a lot of questions. This diagnostic interview may be short or quite long depending on whether your problem is acute or chronic, mild or severe. An effective remedy for an acute condition can be recommended based primarily on the symptoms that are manifesting and a little information about how you cope with illness and who you are as a person. Remedies for serious or chronic conditions are determined after an extensive diagnostic interview. These recommendations are best made by an experienced (not merely trained) homeopath.

The questions will cover a wide range and some may seem wholly unrelated to the problem at hand. For example, a homeopath may ask about your sleep and eating habits, your energy level and emotional states, your mental acuity, and how the weather affects you. There will be questions about the specific character of the illness; for example: Does it start abruptly or come on slowly? Exactly what does it feel like? Are you better or worse at any particular time of day or night? After eating or not eating? Do you have any symptoms in addition to the primary problem—such as nausea or muscle pain with headache? Finally, there will questions about your idiosyncratic reactions to your illness. Some people like to be left alone when they are ill, others prefer company. If you are chilly when sick, do you crave warmth or coolness? Is your appetite affected? Are you demanding or yielding, irritable or placid?

After the interview, the practitioner will consult two references: a Repertory and a Materia Medica. A Repertory is a dictionary of symptoms and illnesses with recommendations for treatment. The Materia Medica is a catalog of the remedies and their effects. The homeopath uses these books to *repertorize,* that is, match your particular array of symptoms to the remedy that resonates with the broadest number of them (*see*: "How to Use This Section" in Part Three, The Materia Medica).

When treating acute illnesses, it isn't necessary to have every symptom detailed in the remedy profile, or even a preponderance of them. In acute care a remedy can help if it overlaps between three and five of your most pressing symptoms. In the case of chronic or severe illness, it is preferable to have a high degree of overlap between the remedy profile and the presenting symptoms. In all cases, the greater the overlap, the more effective the remedy.

If different symptoms come forward in the course of an acute illness, treat the symptoms as they arise. It is not unusual, for example, to use two or more remedies to address the various symptoms throughout a cold, or to use different remedies to treat colds that arise at different times of the year (in homeopathy, a spring cold is different from a winter cold), or that affect different parts of the body in different sequences (a head-to-chest cold, for example, is different from a chest-to-head cold).

TAKING THE CASE

To determine which remedy will be helpful for self-care of an acute illness, ask yourself some or all of the following questions. Make a list of your responses and be as specific as possible with your answers. Compare your symptoms to those listed for the remedies in the Materia Medica (Part Three). The remedy that includes most of your symptoms, or most of your most troubling symptoms, will be the best choice for your particular condition.

1. How did the illness begin? Consider: left or right side, suddenly or gradually, after an injury, from eating or drinking, after exposure to weather (wind, rain, or cold).
2. Scan through your body. What symptoms, if any, are occurring in each area?
3. What are your most pressing symptoms?
4. If there is pain, what does it feel like? Where is it located?
5. If you have a cough, what is it like?
6. Do you have any discharges? If so, describe it (color, odor, consistency, benign or irritating).
7. Do you have a fever? Chills?
8. Are your bowels affected (constipation, diarrhea)?
9. Is your face pale or flushed? If flushed, what color is it (pink, red, purplish)? Are there dark circles under your eyes?
10. What makes you feel better? What makes you feel worse?
11. Is your appetite or thirst affected? Do you crave any foods or drinks? Are you averse to any foods or drinks?
12. Has your sleep pattern changed? How so?
13. Describe your mental state. Consider: ability to concentrate, patience level, alertness, forgetfulness.
14. Has your mood changed? What emotions do you feel most often and most powerfully?
15. Has your energy level changed?

Do I take homeopathic remedies like any other medicine?

Remedies come in several forms. All of them are prepared as lactose-based pellets (sometimes called globules), and some also come as a liquid (sometimes called a tincture). A few remedies—arnica and calendula, for example—are made as creams or gels and are applied topically like any other salve.

When taking pellets or liquids, place the remedy under your tongue. Avoid chewing or swallowing the pellets, you get better absorption if you let them dissolve in your mouth. (This takes a few minutes.)

One dose of a remedy is one to three pellets or three drops of a tincture. Doses are defined by time, not volume; taking one pellet once is the same as taking a handful at once. You don't overdose on the remedy because it is a single dose. If, however, you take one pellet, then let 20 minutes elapse before taking another, you have taken two doses. Repeating doses over time increases the effects of the remedy.

When taking pellets, avoid handling them. Tap them into the cap or onto a piece of paper, then pick up only as many as you need. Pour any extras back into the vial. Handling the pellets can contaminate them. If you put contaminated pellets into the vial, they can alter the entire contents.

When taking homeopathic remedies in any form, avoid strong-smelling substances—mint (toothpaste, food, candies, teas), camphor, or menthol (used in cold remedies and cosmetics)—for 20 to 30 minutes before and after a dose. You should also avoid drinking coffee, black tea, or cola and eating or drinking chocolate for the same amount of time. These substances can negate the effect of the remedy.

Store the remedies in a cool dry place (not the frequently hot and steamy bathroom medicine cabinet). Keep them away from strongly aromatic items, such as perfumes and cosmetics, and any preparations that contain mint, menthol, or camphor.

How often should I take the remedy?

Take the remedies on an as-needed basis, not by a clock-based schedule. Take one dose and wait until you notice an improvement. Do not repeat the dose as long as the improvement continues. When the improvement levels off or subsides, take another dose. The cycle of improvement may be long or short—as short as 10 or 15 minutes—but as long as improvement is under way, additional medication is not needed.

How do I know it's working?

After taking a remedy, one of three things will happen: You will feel better; you will feel worse; or you will feel the same. The reactions depend on whether you have taken a well-chosen remedy.

If you take an appropriate remedy, you will begin to feel better almost immediately. You may feel better mentally or spiritually—more hopeful, for example—before you feel better physically, but feeling better on any level is a sign that the remedy is appropriate to the condition and is working. (If you have taken an appropriate remedy, especially if it is a relatively high potency, you may very quickly fall asleep. When you wake up, you will be greatly improved.)

Another sign that a remedy is working is feeling worse. Remember that homeopathy distinguishes between symptoms and illness, putting symptoms on the side of health. If the symptoms you already have accelerate—a situation that homeopaths call an aggravation—consider it a sign of improvement. Your body's natural defense mechanisms have been strengthened and are fighting the illness. An aggravation, sometimes called a healing crisis, usually passes quickly (within two to three hours), and then you will begin to feel better. An aggravation is usually caused by taking too high a potency. If you get an aggravation, switch to a lower potency of the remedy or take it less frequently.

You can have both reactions at once: believing that you are getting better even though your symptoms are aggravated. This is an example of Hering's laws of cure (*see:* Hering's Laws of Cure), feeling better at a deep level (your mental or spiritual self) while feeling worse closer to the surface (your physical symptoms) is also a sign of improvement.

If, however, you take an inappropriate remedy, you will also feel worse, or no better on any level. The difference here is that your symptoms don't abate after about two hours of taking the remedy. If this happens, try another remedy.

Stay with one remedy for as long as it helps. Change to another remedy only if the first one is ineffective or after it stops creating improvement.

HERING'S LAWS OF CURE

Dr. Constantine Hering (1800–1880), a German physician who is considered the father of American Homeopathy, observed that illness resolves in predictable stages. In the mid-1800s, he codified these observations into three principles that are used to gauge the general progress of healing.

1. Symptoms resolve in the reverse order from which they appeared.
2. Symptoms resolve from top to bottom (head to feet).
3. Symptoms resolve in more important organs first, followed by less important organs.

Are there any side effects?

It is not entirely true that homeopathy has no side effects. Homeopathy arose through a series of clinical trials, or *provings,* in which symptoms of illnesses were deliberately created in healthy people. If you choose an inappropriate remedy, you may find yourself doing a proving, that is, you may develop symptoms that the remedy is capable of eliciting in addition to the symptoms you already have. The symptoms generated in a proving are transient, but they are real and may be uncomfortable while they are manifesting.

Over and above that, however, Hahnemann rejected the idea that you can acknowledge some effects of a remedy and dismiss others. An assessment of the totality of symptoms is a cornerstone of homeopathic philosophy, and so all effects, even those that another treatment system might discount as "side" effects, are accepted as part of the remedy picture and acknowledged as desirable in some cases.

Can I use homeopathy if I am taking other medicines?

Dr. Hahnemann was opposed to mixing therapies. However, the standard medical practices in place in his lifetime included radical and harmful procedures such as bloodletting, purging and fasting, and medicines derived from toxic chemicals such as arsenic and mercury.

Contemporary practitioners are more lenient. Combining therapies can be very effective, with a few caveats. Be sure you have proper supervision from trained and experienced people. Stay alert to your condition and keep everyone informed of your progress. Avoid combining so many practices that it becomes difficult to sort out what is useful. Drop practices that do not help and, especially, drop ones that are harmful.

Whether used alone or as a complement to standard medical treatments, homeopathy can speed healing—safely, rapidly, deeply, gently, and effectively—in a wide variety of illnesses and injuries.

PART TWO

BACK AND NECK PAIN

FREQUENTLY ASKED QUESTIONS

Why does my back hurt?

A variety of factors contribute to back pain. Injuries and weak trunk muscles are implicated in about 80 percent of backaches. Obesity, which shifts the center of gravity forward, places stress on the spine which can cause or exacerbate pain. Smoking reduces the amount of oxygen in your blood which diminishes nutrition to the tissues and can also contribute to a painful back.

Age and heredity also play a role. Absent an injury, back pain tends to arise in people between the ages of 30 and 55, partly as a result of the natural wear and tear on the spine. (Not all degeneration causes pain, however, which can make a diagnosis difficult.) The risk of pain tends to diminish for men past age 50; however, it increases for women due to the onset and progress of osteoporosis. There is some evidence that intervertebral disk disease and herniated disk problems run in families.

Occupational hazards, such as physically heavy work (frequent lifting, bending, or twisting), static work postures (prolonged sitting or standing in one position), and repetitive work such as assembly line operations are the most prevalent contributing factors. People who drive motorized vehicles for four or more hours a day are three times as likely to develop herniated disks as other people. Sitting exerts pressure on the disks in the lower back; the force has been estimated as 50 percent greater than when you stand. This pressure combined with the persistent vibration from the motor can accelerate disk problems.

Your emotional health plays a role as well. Back pain can cause depression, pain and depression lead to diminished activity, diminished activity can aggravate back pain.

WHEN TO SEE A DOCTOR

Most backache is transitory and resolves without intervention within two months. If your pain is severe, lasts longer than two months, or is the result of an accident or injury, it is best to have it evaluated by a physician.

See a Doctor Immediately If . . .

- you get a backache after an injury.
- you have a severe back pain and an unexplained fever.
- you have a backache that comes on gradually and worsens slowly, with stiff back, neck, legs, and fever.

See a Doctor If . . .

- your back pain has not resolved within three to eight weeks.
- you have back pain that is persistent or recurrent and incapacitating.
- you have trouble urinating.
- you have pain or weakness in one or both legs.
- you have severe back pain, sudden weight loss, and pain elsewhere in your body.
- in addition to back pain, your joints ache and swell.

Are backaches a symptom of an underlying illness?

Backache may accompany inflammatory illnesses such as arthritis, a systemic infection such as a cold or flu, a kidney or bladder infection, and stomach disorders such as an ulcer or pancreatic inflammation. Pain that persists after the infection resolves should be evaluated by a doctor.

Cancer in the spine is extremely rare—fewer than 1 in 10,000 people with back pain have tumors of the spine. Spinal tumors that do occur usually result from cancer that originates in another part of the body and metastasizes to the back.

Why doesn't my doctor understand how much this hurts?

Your doctor does understand that you hurt. But because pain perception has emotional as well as physical components, it cannot be measured in absolute terms the same way that, for example, the stages of healing for a broken bone can be measured. Pain is always relative and its perception depends on two factors: *pain threshold* and *pain tolerance.*

Pain threshold is simply the level of stimulus—how much pressure—that is needed for the sensation to be felt and interpreted as pain. This may be reflexive and almost instantaneous, as when you jerk your hand away from a hot surface or leap back from a loud noise, or it may be gradual, as when pain from an infected tooth grows and grows.

Pain tolerance, on the other hand, is a term for the idiosyncratic way each of us interprets the sensation and severity of pain. This varies from person to person and, oftentimes, within the same person. Some people can rest relatively contentedly after major surgery and never want pain medication; others are so debilitated by any pain that they need an anesthetic to have a splinter removed.

Since the perception of pain is so idiosyncratic, it can be more perplexing than illuminating in medical philosophies that look for universal standards and solutions.

How is the approach to diagnosis different in homeopathy?

A homeopath will be very interested in how you perceive and describe the pain you experience. A crushing pain (pressing inward) is significantly different from one that is bursting (pressing out). A pain on the left side takes a different remedy from one on the right side. Pain that starts on the left and moves to the right is different from one that is localized. Time and weather are also important. Night pain is different from day pain. Pain brought on by or worsened by cold, heat, humidity, or wind is treated differently from pains that are relieved or eradicated by those conditions.

When you consult a homeopath, he will ask you a series of very detailed questions about yourself, your life and habits, and your ailment. (This diagnostic interview is called *taking the case.*) Many of the questions will be the same or similar to those that a doctor would ask: When did the pain start? How long does it last? Are you taking anything for it? Is it helping? Is the pain generalized or localized? Have you noticed whether it starts after you eat certain foods?

In addition to these kinds of questions, a homeopath will you ask about your mental and emotional state— both when you are in the throes of a backache and when you are not. She may ask: Are you alert or forgetful? Do your moods shift or are they stable? Do you want to be left alone when you don't feel well or do you prefer company? Additional questions will cover your eating habits; sleep and dream patterns; and your level of contentment with your job, your family, and your social life.

Don't try to outguess the therapist. In order to recommend an effective homeopathic remedy, the therapist must have accurate information. It is not in your best interest to claim that you are sensitive, laugh and cry easily, and feel better walking outdoors in a light breeze when in fact you prefer to be indoors, would rather die than cry, and tend to be sarcastic. However much you may wish that you fit a particular description or believe that it is more desirable to be a certain way, misinformation will lead to misdiagnosis. There are no wrong answers in the quest for health.

What can I do to combat backaches?

Transient backaches are usually the result of strain from lifting (especially if you twisted or turned while lifting), poor posture, an injury, or from an inflammatory illness. Become aware of how you inhabit your body and learn to sit, stand, and move in ways that minimize the possibility of injuring your back. Keep a record of your backaches and try to identify whether there are patterns of onset that you can change or avoid.

Practice consistent moderate exercise that strengthens your back. A program that includes walking, strength training, and stretching is a good all-around preventative for backache. Talk to your doctor about which exercises would be suitable for you. If you want to work with a trainer at a gym, be sure that person understands your goals and is sensitive to your needs. Gung-ho workouts can do more harm than good.

Chronic backache often involves structural damage or

anomalies or an illness such as osteoporosis. See your internist and have some basic checkups to try to identify the cause of the pain. Examine your family's medical history. There is some evidence that susceptibility to particular back problems—intervertebral disk disease and herniated disks, for example—as well as to inflammatory illnesses, such as arthritis, tend to run in families. You can't change a genetic predisposition to an illness, but the information is helpful in diagnosis and treatment.

Are there medical tests to diagnose backaches?

Back pain of less than two months duration is commonly diagnosed by your description of your symptoms, observation of your gait and posture, your medical history, and a physical exam. If these fail to identify the problem, additional tests, such as X-rays, a CAT scan, or an MRI may be undertaken to identify what is causing or aggravating the pain.

The diagnostic tests fall into three general categories: imaging tests that examine bones and muscles, neurological tests that evaluate the functioning of your nerves, and blood tests to confirm or rule out various illnesses, such as arthritis or gout. The imaging tests include X-rays, MRIs, CAT (or CT) scans, myelograms, and bone scans. The primary neurological tests are EMG (electromyography) and nerve conduction tests. The blood tests are the familiar ones from your annual physical: blood count, blood chemistry, and ESR (Erythrocyte Sedimentation Rate). There are special blood tests to diagnose arthritis.

IMAGING TESTS

Pictures of the structures of your back are invaluable in diagnosing the causes of back pain. A variety of tests, from simple X-rays to X-rays enhanced with sophisticated computer technology, have evolved over the decades. The main tests, their uses and limitations, and some cautions are described here.

X-rays. Although less accurate than other imaging techniques because the density of the body tends to create shadows in the image, X-rays are helpful in diagnosing bone diseases, such as arthritis, degenerative disk disease, osteoporosis, and cancer as well as injuries or structural anomalies such as fractures, bone spurs, curvature, and spondylolisthesis. X-rays are not useful for diagnosing sciatica or muscle injuries. Fractures of the vertebra's back plate (caused by compression) often do not show up on standard X-rays.

In diagnosing lower back pain, your doctor will typically ask for five X-rays of your lumbar spine taken with you standing upright: one front to back, one from each side, and two oblique (angled) views. Additional views taken while you bend forward or backward may also be helpful.

MRI (Magnetic Resonance Imaging). Often used as a follow-up to X-rays, this system uses a magnetic field rather than radiation to generate pictures of the intervertebral disks and nerve roots. The test itself is painless, but some people find the environment of the test unsettling. The machine makes a noise similar to a jackhammer (although not as loud), you must lie still in a tube not much larger than your body, which some people find claustrophobic, and the test usually lasts for about 45 minutes. An MRI will aid the diagnosis of a disk and nerve problems such as sciatica, herniated disks, tumors, and spinal cord disease. It is not useful for diagnosing bone injuries and abnormalities

CAUTION: People with artificial heart valves, pacemakers, or metal clips should not be subjected to MRI. Also, the test may be enhanced by using contrast dyes, which are injected into the patient. Some of these dyes contain iodine. A dye-enhanced test is contraindicated if you are allergic to iodine or shellfish.

Myelography. An enhanced X-ray procedure, in which an iodine-based dye is injected into the fluid in the spinal canal. The dye highlights anomalies so that they can show up on an X-ray. This test may be followed by CT scans to give the physician a clear picture of the relationship between bone and nerves. Myelography is useful for the evaluation of complicated disk problems, pinched nerves, and compressive abnormalities such as stenosis.

CAUTION: Myelography is contraindicated in patients who are allergic to iodine or shellfish.

CAT scan. Sometimes called a CT scan, CAT scans are similar to an X-ray, except that the area being examined is smaller. CAT is the acronym for *computerized axial tomography.* "Tomography" is radiography (X-raying) without shadows. "Axial" refers to the narrow cross sections that are taken from a particular axis, or direction, and "computerized" means that a computer is part of the equipment.

During a CAT scan, a narrow X-ray beam takes a picture of a cross-section of your back and maps the bones, muscles, organs, tissues, and fluids. The technician may take about a dozen of these pictures, each one taking one or two seconds to complete. The images are fed into a computer that translates them into black, white, and gray tones, and are printed out. Your doctor will analyze the images for abnormalities that suggest disease. CAT scans are helpful in the examination of intervertebral disks.

CAT scans do not interfere with pacemakers or other cardiac appliances.

Bone scan. Rather than using iodine-based dyes, a bone scan uses an injected radioactive isotope to identify inflammation, infection, osteoporosis, and cancer. The isotope collects in greater amounts in areas of abnormal bone. The test may be targeted (localized) or throughout the skeleton. You must lie flat for the entire procedure; a test of the entire skeleton takes about four hours.

NEUROLOGICAL TESTS

These tests help your doctor determine if there is damage to a nerve or muscle and, if there is, to identify which nerve or muscle is involved.

EMG (electromyography). This test measures whether a muscle is receiving too much, too little, or just enough stimulation from the nerve. Usually the leg muscles are tested, and the test consists of two parts: recordings of the changes in the electrical state on the skin and in the muscle.

To test the surface response, electrodes are placed on the skin over a muscle. The muscle is stimulated and an oscilloscope records the changes in the electrical state. The test in repeated along the course of the muscle and its nerve. The rate at which the changes occur indicates how well the nerve is functioning. To test the muscle's response, a recording needle is inserted into the muscle, and readings are taken with the muscle at rest and when active.

EMG tests are helpful in identifying which nerve roots may be affected by a herniated disk or other spinal abnormality.

Nerve conduction tests. These tests measure the speed at which an impulse travels from the nerve to the muscle. A slower than normal speed suggests an injury to the nerve.

BLOOD TESTS

Since most backache arises from mechanical causes—injuries to the muscles or bones—blood tests are not usually required. However, they are helpful in diagnosing backache that arises due to infections or inflammatory illnesses.

Blood count. Literally a count of the various kinds of cells present in your blood, this test is useful for determining anemia (decreased number of red blood cells) and infections (increased number of white blood cells).

Blood chemistry. A measure of the concentration of the various chemical and mineral components in your blood. This screening test is especially helpful for diagnosing kidney and liver problems (including gout) and metabolic disorders.

ESR, or Erythrocyte (red blood cell) Sedimentation Rate. This test indicates the presence of inflammation or infection. It may be followed by additional tests to identify arthritis.

Is a medical diagnosis helpful to a homeopath?

Any information you have about your condition is helpful. Hundreds of remedies have been developed over the centurys since homeopathy began. Each remedy fits a particular constellation of symptoms and many of the remedy profiles are long and detailed. A medical diagnosis, such as arthritis or a herniated disk, coupled with the specific information you provide about your particular condition, will help your homeopath identify an appropriate remedy more quickly.

How are backaches categorized?

Backaches fall into two broad categories: acute (or transient) and chronic. Acute backaches generally arise from sprain, strain, or spasm caused by injury or overexertion, accompany an acute illness such as a cold or the flu, or are part of a flare-up of a chronic illness such as arthritis. The pain usually resolves itself within two months with rest. When backache accompanies illness, the pain resolves as the illness resolves. Chronic backache, on the other hand, may be related to degeneration, injury, congenital anomalies (such as curvatures or abnormal bone formations), or a chronic illness.

Whether acute or chronic, backaches are further classified by the area of the back that is affected—for example, arthritis in the neck is called cervical spondylitis—or, as in the case of vertebral or disk problems, by the name of the particular bone or structure that is involved. The vertebrae of the spine are divided into five sections: 7 cervical (neck) bones, 12 thoracic (chest), 5 lumbar (lower back), the sacrum (composed of 5 fused bones), and the coccyx (composed of 4 fused bones). The vertebrae are numbered from top to bottom beginning with "1" in each section; thus, the cervical vertebrae are C1 through C7, the thoracic are T1 through T12, and so on.

Finally, certain backaches are due to specific illnesses. When this is the case, the name of the illness is the name of the backache. Ankylosing spondylitis, for example, is a particular form of arthritis that affects the spine. Similarly, lumbago, although not a specific illness, is a common term for nonspecific generalized low back pain.

How can I tell what kind of backache I have?

Onset, persistence, and severity are the measures of whether you have an acute or potentially chronic problem. A backache that has a vague origin, is especially painful, or does not get better within two months should be evaluated by a doctor.

Any injury to your head, neck, or back should be considered a medical emergency. The side effects of head and neck trauma in particular can be crippling or fatal. It is better to be a little embarrassed about overreacting than risk the possible consequences from an undiagnosed injury.

DEFINING BACKACHE

Injury

Injuries are usually memorable and therefore relatively easy to diagnose. Muscles are highly specialized, usually one muscle performs one action. For example, your biceps muscle allows you to bend your elbow; the triceps muscle allows you to straighten it. This specialization helps your doctor identify which muscle is injured: If you have pain during a specific movement, the muscle that performs that movement is injured.

Backache from strain, sprain, spasm, or overexertion will usually resolve within two months. In the first 48 hours, back strains and sprains can be treated as you would any other sprain: with rest, ice, and compression. After 48 hours, the injury will respond better to heat and gentle motion.

CAUTION: Persistent pain that follows an injury, especially an injury to the head, neck, or back must be evaluated by a physician. Undiagnosed internal damage may be crippling or fatal.

OVEREXERTION: STRAIN, SPRAIN, SPASM

The most common backaches are strains and sprains due to overexertion, or from *torque,* twisting or turning especially if the torque occurred while lifting. Impact, such as from falling, being struck, or a car accident may also cause strain or torque injuries to muscles, bones, or connective tissue.

Muscle spasm may occur independently of an injury. It may arise as a reflex reaction if nerves are stimulated by an underlying condition such as a herniated disk or bone deformity. Spasm may also affect uninjured muscles near an injured muscle due to *splinting.* Splinting is the instinctive contracting of healthy muscles around an injured muscle to hold it still and avoid pain or to compensate for reduced range of movement.

If your backache is due to strain, sprain, spasm, or overexertion, you will have some or all of these symptoms:

Onset: Follows trauma.

Sensation: Aching, bruised sensation. Numbness, tingling. Pain during specific motions.

Modalities

Worse: Motion. Pressure. Cold, damp weather. Drafts.

Better: Rest. Gentle motion as injury heals. Moist or dry heat.

Concomitants: Bruising. Swelling.

Homeopathic remedies that may be helpful for backache due to injuries include:

Aesculus hippocastanum. Agaricus muscarius. Argentum metallicum. Arnica. Bryonia. Calcarea carbonica. Causticum. Cimicifuga racemosa. Gelsemium. Graphites. Hypericum. Kali carbonicum. Nux vomica. Phosphorus. Pulsatilla. Rhus toxicodendron. Sepia. Silica.

WHIPLASH

A controversial diagnosis, whiplash results from either hyperextension or hyperflexion of the cervical vertebrae. In layman's terms, this means having your neck snapped back and/or forth, usually as a result of impact in a car accident.

The symptoms of whiplash are pain and stiffness in the neck. The pain may radiate to the shoulders and arms.

If you suffer with whiplash, you will have some or all of these symptoms:

Onset: Follows trauma.

Sensation: Pain. Stiffness. Numbness, tingling.

Modalities

   Worse: Motion. Cold, damp weather. Drafts.

   Better: Rest. Moist or dry heat.

Concomitants: Pain in shoulders and arms. Tingling and numbness in arms and hands.

Homeopathic remedies that may be helpful for whiplash include:

Aesculus hippocastanum. Arnica. Belladonna. Berberis vulgaris. Bryonia. Calcarea carbonica. Causticum. Cimicifuga racemosa. Eupatorium perfoliatum. Gelsemium. Graphites. Hypericum. Lycopodium. Nux vomica. Pulsatilla. Silica. Sulphur.

Pinched nerves

Your spine is a housing for your spinal cord, the main trunk of your nerves. Every nerve in your body has its root in the spine. Between each pair of vertebrae are exit channels for the nerve fibers. If there are any anomalies within the spinal canal or in the size of the channels due to changes in the size or shape of the bone or the disks, pressure is exerted on the nerve and pain results. A common cause of this kind of nerve pain is a herniated disk. Any disk can herniate, but the most common sites are in the neck and lower back. Another common nerve impingement backache is sciatica, which takes its name from the particular nerve involved.

HERNIATED DISK

Sometimes called a ruptured or slipped disk, herniation is a break in the disk's cartilaginous shell that allows the jellylike core to protrude and exert pressure on the nerve. The rupture may result from an injury or from degeneration due to illness, overuse, or aging. The most common cause is the "lift with a twist"—in some cases simply bending and then lifting the weight of your body can be sufficient to cause an injury.

If you have a herniated disk, you will have some or all of these symptoms:

Onset: Sudden. May follow an injury.

Sensation: Sharp, severe, shooting pain. Localized pain. Pain that follows a specific track.

Modalities

Worse: Movement.

Better: Still. Moist or dry heat.

Concomitants: Muscle spasm, splinting. Weakness, numbness, pins and needles. Coldness. Pain and weakness may extend to legs or arms.

Mentals and Generals: Bored, restless, feels there is "nothing to do."

Homeopathic remedies that may be helpful for herniated disks include:

Agaricus muscarius. Causticum. Colocynthis. Hypericum. Rhus toxicodendron.

DEGENERATED DISK

As you age, your intervertebral disks may dehydrate and become smaller, less resilient, and less effective at absorbing shock. Some calcification may occur; in rare cases, a bony fusion forms across the disk. Tiny bone spurs, called *osteophytes*, may develop on the vertebrae and narrow the disk space. Although all disks degenerate over time, some are painful and others are not.

Typically, this condition affects people in their 40s. Symptoms include back pain alone or back and leg or arm pain. The remedies suggested for herniated disk can be used for degenerated disks as well.

SCIATICA

The sciatic nerve exits the spine at the sacrum, travels across the back of the hip and down the leg where it branches into a network of smaller and smaller nerves. A herniated lumbar disk is often implicated in sciatic pain, but the pain may occur without disk damage. If your doctor suspects sciatica, she will test your reflexes at the knee and ankle and may perform a straight leg test. In this test, the doctor supports your leg and moves it through its range of motion. Unfortunately, this movement can be painful, but the specificity of when the pain occurs as your leg is moved helps in the diagnosis.

Spondylolisthesis and Piriformis syndrome, discussed below, mimic sciatica.

If you suffer with sciatica, you will have some or all of these symptoms:

Sensation: Severe and incapacitating pain in lower back and legs. Shooting pain. Pain that follows a specific track. Pain, weakness, numbness that extends to the legs.

Modalities
   Worse: Coughing, sneezing, or straining at stool.
     Bending or twisting.
   Better: Still. Moist or dry heat.
Concomitants: Numbness or abnormal sensitivity, tingling, or "pins and needles" in the leg. Odd gait.

Homeopathic remedies that may be helpful for sciatica include:
   Berberis vulgaris. Bryonia. Calcarea carbonica. Colocynthis. Hypericum. Kali carbonicum. Pulsatilla. Rhus toxicodendron. Sepia. Silica. Sulphur.
   left-sided: Causticum.
   right-sided: Lycopodium.

Spondylolisthesis
From the Greek *spondylos*, spine, and *oblisthesis*, a slipping, spondylolisthesis is a condition in which the lower lumbar vertebrae slip out of position over the sacrum by sliding forward (toward the abdomen). It results from two causes: either degeneration or as an overuse injury due to heavy lifting and/or throwing. The slippage results when repeated stress accumulates and causes a fatigue break, a fracture, in the lower spine. Diabetics are prone to degenerative spondylolisthesis. Particular athletes—gymnasts, interior linemen in football, weight lifters, javelin throwers, and sumo wrestlers—are prone to spondylolisthesis from overuse injuries. In either case, the symptoms are similar to those of sciatica—severe, shooting pain along the track of either or both sciatic nerves and the condition is diagnosed with bone scans and X-rays.

   The remedies recommended for sciatica, in particular Sulphur, can be helpful for spondylolisthesis.

Piriformis syndrome

This syndrome results from wearing tight jeans and carrying a wallet in your back pocket. Pressure from the clothing and wallet is transferred to the piriformis muscle, a muscle deep in your buttocks, close to the bone. The muscle goes into spasm and presses on the sciatic nerve; the overstimulated nerve sends pain shooting across your back and down your legs.

The immediate solution to the problem is to relax the spasmed muscle. Heat, gentle stretching, and relief from the aggravating cause will accomplish this. The long-term solution is prevention by wearing looser clothing.

SPINAL STENOSIS

The symptoms of spinal stenosis are similar to those of a herniated disk: back and leg pain, numbness and a burning sensation in both legs, weakness, coldness, or pins and needles. Stenosis, however, is a narrowing of the spinal canal, the housing of the spinal cord, due to bone spurs or deformities resulting from degeneration, swollen joints, displaced ligaments, or thickening of the *lamina,* the vertebrae's thin bony plates. The narrowed canal presses on the nerves inside it. Stenosis generally affects people who are over 50, although some people have a congenitally narrow canal.

Spinal stenosis generally gets worse over time and is diagnosed by your medical and family history, a physical exam, and imaging tests including X-rays, CAT scan, myelography, and MRI.

If you suffer with spinal stenosis, you will have some or all of these symptoms:

Onset: After age 50.

Sensation: Back and leg pain. Numbness and burning sensation in both legs. Weakness, numbness, coldness, or pins and needles.

Modalities

> *Worse:* When walking downhill or on a level surface. Coughing, sneezing or straining at stool. Pain persists while resting.
>
> *Better:* Rest. Leaning forward. Walking uphill. Squatting or sitting, lying on side.

Homeopathic remedies that may be helpful for spinal stenosis include:

Agaricus muscarius. Berberis vulgaris. Bryonia. Calcarea carbonica. Causticum. Colocynthis. Hypericum. Kali carbonicum. Lycopodium Pulsatilla. Rhus toxicodendron. Sepia. Silica. Sulphur.

Inflammatory illnesses

Inflammation, literally "to flame within," is defined by four factors: redness, heat, swelling, and pain. It is a defensive reaction in which your blood vessels dilate, resulting in swelling intended to isolate the injury or pathogens (germs) and pain to remind you to hold still and not injure yourself any further. The redness and heat come from increased circulation as your blood cells work to repair the damage or kill the intruders. (Body heat comes from the friction of your blood cells against the vessel walls.)

This defensive activity can feel like an illness in and of itself, and particular kinds of inflammation define certain diseases. Illnesses that end in "itis"—arthritis, sinusitis, appendicitis, hepatitis—are inflammatory diseases. Body aches, loss of appetite, and generalized discomfort are typical concomitants of inflammation.

Spondylitis

From *spondylos,* Greek for vertebra, and *itis,* inflammation, spondylitis is a form of degenerative arthritis that primarily affects the joints between the vertebrae. It is associated with aging and the normal wear and tear on the back over time. Cervical spondylitis affects the neck, ankylosing spondylitis affects the entire spine and may include the sacroiliac joint.

As with other degenerative conditions, the symptoms may be relatively subtle or severe and debilitating. The symptoms include limited mobility with pain at the extreme range of motion and pain or stiffness that is worse in the morning and in cold damp weather. Generally, the person is worse after sitting; riding in motor vehicles (cars, trains) may be intolerable. Lifting, twisting, or bending is impossible because of the pain. A back brace or neck collar, regular gentle exercise, and weight maintenance can help relieve pain.

Spondylitis is diagnosed by history and imaging tests. X-rays should be taken to determine the presence of bony spurs, called *osteophytes,* and/or minor bone deformities. The spurs contribute to the stiffening.

Ankylosing spondylitis

Ankyl means stiffen and *-osis* is a condition, so ankylosing spondylitis literally means a condition in which an inflamed spine stiffens. A form of rheumatoid arthritis, it is intensely painful and usually affects men. It may begin when a man is in his 20s or 30s, and the first attack is often mistaken for a pulled muscle. The sacroiliac joint may also become inflamed and cause pain in the hip as well as the back.

The symptoms of ankylosing spondylitis include low back pain and referred pain to the hips and legs. The joints between the thoracic spine and the ribs may become stiff and restrict breathing. With stiff joints in the neck and upper spine, the person may walk hunched over or crouched, which may become a permanent deformity.

Ankylosing spondylitis is diagnosed with X-rays and blood tests.

If you suffer with ankylosing spondylitis, you will have some or all of these symptoms:

Sensation: Stiffness. Intense pain.

Modalities

> *Worse:* In the morning. Cold damp weather. From sitting or riding in motor vehicles. Sitting and rising from sitting.

> *Better:* Standing. Gentle consistent exercise.

Concomitants: Headache. Pain in hips or legs. Weakness.

Mentals and Generals: Lifting, twisting, or bending is impossible because of the pain. Limited mobility with pain at the extreme range of motion.

Homeopathic remedies that may be helpful for ankylosing spondylitis include:

Aesculus hippocastanum. Agaricus muscarius. Argentum metallicum. Berberis vulgaris. Bryonia. Calcarea carbonica. Causticum. Colocynthis. Gelsemium. Phosphorus. Pulsatilla. Silica. Sulphur.

Cervical spondylitis

In cervical spondylitis, bony deposits form on the neck portion of the spine. These deposits inhibit motion and can impinge on the nerves, causing severe pain. To compensate, you may "splint" your neck—that is, you will try to hold your head very still, and the muscle tension from splinting may increase the pain.

Symptoms of cervical spondylitis include pain or weakness in the arms, numbness or weakness in the hands, and increased clumsiness. It is diagnosed with a physical examination and imaging tests including X-rays, myelogram, CAT scan, or MRI.

If you suffer with cervical spondylitis, you will have some or all of these symptoms:

Location: Neck, shoulder, arm, and hand pain.

Sensation: Severe pain. Stiffness. Weakness.

Modalities

   Worse: Movement. Cold, damp weather. Drafts.

   Better: Still. Heat.

Concomitants: Headache. An odd gait. Increased clumsiness. Weakness, numbness, or tingling in the hands.

Homeopathic remedies that may be helpful for cervical spondylitis include:

Aesculus hippocastanum. Agaricus muscarius. Arnica. Belladonna. Berberis vulgaris. Bryonia. Calcarea carbonica. Causticum. Cimicifuga racemosa. Colocynthis. Eupatorium perfoliatum. Gelsemium. Graphites. Hypericum. Kali carbonicum. Lycopodium. Nux vomica. Pulsatilla. Rhus toxicodendron. Sepia. Silica. Sulphur.

ARTHRITIS

Perhaps the most prevalent joint disease, arthritis has two broad forms: *osteoarthritis,* usually considered noninflammatory, and *rheumatoid,* or inflammatory. All forms of arthritis exhibit the defining symptoms of inflammation—swelling, redness, heat, and pain—in one or more joints, as well as stiffness relieved by gentle motion. In osteoarthritis, a distinctive cracking noise called *crepitus* is common. Health organizations estimate that more than one-third of all Americans are affected by some form of arthritis. The disease is associated with aging and affects more women than men. Arthritis usually begins in weight-bearing joints such as hip, knee, and foot joints, and in joints that are frequently active, such as the wrists and fingers. In extreme cases, hip or knee replacement surgery is recommended.

Osteoarthritis is present in about 10 percent of the population, many of whom have no symptoms. It is a degenerative and noninflammatory condition in which the cushioning layer of cartilage between the bones of a joint is eroded. Cysts and osteophytes, small bone growths and spurs, develop around the margins of the joint. Osteoarthritis often occurs in the neck, lower back, and hips. It is exacerbated by obesity. Pain arises from the growths, which impede movement, and from bare bone rubbing against bare bone. Osteoarthritis is diagnosed by your medical and family history, your symptoms, and X-rays.

Rheumatoid arthritis is the most common inflammatory joint disease. It has a sudden onset, may be chronic or intermittent, and produces a characteristic deformity that can be crippling. It usually afflicts knee, hand, and wrist joints, but can also affect the hips and lumbar spine. Overt symptoms of joint pain and stiffness may be preceded or accompanied by tiredness and feeling generally unwell. The symptoms are usually worse in the morning. Rheumatoid arthritis is diagnosed by your medical and family history, your symptoms, X-rays, and a special blood test to identify rheumatoid factor.

If you suffer with backaches from arthritis, you will have some or all of these symptoms:

Sensation: Deep aching. Joints, stiff, red, hot, swollen.
Modalities
  Worse: In the morning. After resting.
  Better: Movement, consistent gentle exercise. Heat.
Concomitants: Fatigue. Frustration.

Homeopathic remedies that may be helpful for arthritic backaches include:
  Neck: Arnica. Belladonna. Berberis vulgaris. Bryonia.

Calcarea carbonica. Causticum. Cimifuga racemosa. Eupatorium perfoliatum. Gelsemium. Graphites. Hypericum. Nux vomica. Pulsatilla. Silica. Sulphur.

Lower back: Aesculus hippocastanum. Agaricus muscari. Belladonna. Berberis vulgaris. Bryonia. Causticum. Cimicifuga racemosa. Colocynthis. Gelsemium. Graphites. Hypericum. Kali carbonicum. Lycopodium. Pulsatilla. Phosphorus. Rhus toxicodendron. Sepia. Sulphur. Zinc.

FIBROMYALGIA

Sometimes called fibromyositis or myofascial pain, fibromyalgia is a condition in which pain arises from inflamed muscles, muscle fibers, or the myofascial sheath, the membrane that surrounds the muscles. It is difficult to diagnose and treat effectively. Fibromyalgia generally affects the upper back, shoulders, and shoulder blades. It is characterized by referred pain, that is, pressure on a ''trigger point'' will elicit pain in another area, and frequently is accompanied by depression.

Fibromyalgia is diagnosed by your medical, personal, and family history and by tests to rule out other causes. It responds well to antidepressive treatments, massage, consistent gentle exercise, and heat.

If you suffer with fibromyalgia, you will have some or all of these symptoms:

Sensation: Stiffness. Deep aching. Referred pain.

Modalities

Better: Movement. Heat.

Concomitants: Depression. Frustration. Passivity.

Homeopathic remedies that may be helpful for fibromyalgia include:

Aesculus hippocastanum. Belladonna. Bryonia. Calcarea carbonica. Causticum. Gelsemium. Graphites. Hypericum. Lycopodium. Kali carbonicum. Nux vomica. Phosphorus. Pulsatilla. Sepia. Sulphur. Zinc.

Osteoporosis and osteomalacia

Osteoporosis is not a specific illness, rather it is a general term for an array of illnesses that result in a loss of bone mass that compromises the bone's ability to provide support. The weakened bone is prone to spontaneous fractures. Any bone may be affected, but the vertebrae in the lower thoracic and lumbar spine are most often affected.

The condition affects more women than men and is most prevalent in postmenopausal women. It is associated with aging and with diminished nutrition, particularly of calcium and vitamin D.

Osteomalacia, the adult form of rickets, is frequently implicated in osteoporosis. From the Greek *osteon,* bone, and *malakia,* softening, the condition is characterized by increasing softness of the bones to the point where they are brittle, flexible, and prone to deformity. Its symptoms include rheumatic pains in the pelvis, limbs, trunk, and chest, anemia, and progressive weakness.

Medical treatments include supplements of calcium, fluorides, and vitamin D, a program of consistent low-impact exercise such as walking, and strengthening exercise such as weight training or swimming. Sunlight helps your body metabolize vitamin D, so exercising outdoors provides added benefit. Postmenopausal women often benefit from hormone replacement therapy.

Homeopathic remedies that may be helpful for osteoporosis include:

Argentum metallicum. Calcarea carbonica. Lycopodium. Silica.

THE DIAGNOSTIC INTERVIEW

Whether you see a doctor, a homeopath, or both, the more specific you can be about your condition, the better they will be able to help you. The following questions are typical of what a doctor will ask. A homeopath will also want information about your specific reaction to your condition (*see*: "Taking the Case" in Part One).

When did the pain start?
Do some actions make the pain worse?
Do you have symptoms involving your legs or bladder?
Do you have pain in the thigh or buttocks?
Do you have numbness in your legs?
Do you have trouble moving your legs?
Are your bowels and bladder functioning normally?
When you change positions, does the pain change?
Do you have any other medical problems?
Do you have high blood pressure, coronary artery disease, or any other disease involving a major organ system?
Have you ever had complications of atherosclerosis such as stroke or chest pain?

Are you allergic to any medications?
Do you smoke?
Do you drink alcohol regularly? What kind and how much?
Does your job require heavy lifting, or are you mostly sedentary at work?
Are repetitive motions part of doing your job?

PART THREE

THE MATERIA MEDICA, A CATALOG OF REMEDIES

HOW TO USE THIS SECTION

The following section is the *Materia Medica* (Latin for "Materials of Medicine"). It is a catalog of 25 remedies demonstrated to be helpful for various kinds of back and neck pain. In this book the Materia Medica is divided into two sections; the information in each section is essentially the same, but it is organized differently. The classic homeopathic references describe the remedies in narrative lists arranged by category (location, sensation, modalities, etc.), and you'll find that here as well. However, when trying to decide between two remedies it can be helpful to be able to compare the descriptions side by side, and so the information is also given in chart form. An additional diagnostic chart helps you narrow down the remedies that are helpful for stiffness, weakness, or pain in different areas of the back.

Each remedy description follows the same format. At the top of the page is the full name of the remedy, its common name, and its official abbreviation. Below the remedy name is a list of symptoms divided into specific categories that help in deciding which to choose for a particular condition. The categories are:

Helpful for: A list of the kinds of back and neck pain for which the remedy can be used.

Sensation: Where the pain localizes, how it moves, and the specific sensations you might feel. Typical descriptions include: dull, aching, or shooting; stiffness or weakness; burning or chills; flying pains, dragging pain, or waves of pain.

Modalities: What makes you or your symptoms feel better? What makes you or your symptoms feel worse?

Concomitants: These are symptoms that you may experience in addition to the backache, for example, pain that extends to your legs or that radiates into your abdomen, stiff neck with headache, trembling, awkward gait.

Mentals & Generals: These are symptoms such as forgetfulness or confusion, changes in your emotional state (irritable, whiny, desires solitude, desires company), and alterations in your sleep patterns or appetite (food cravings or aversions).

A short summary follows each list. The summary highlights the characteristic symptoms of a particular remedy, the kind of personality structure that usually matches the remedy, and information to help you decide between remedies with similar profiles. Homeopathy often uses metaphor and descriptive comparisons—pain may be described as "like a thousand little hammers" or "like lightning," or may cause a patient to "den up like a bear," or symptoms may erupt "volcanically." These images are intended to give an accurate and recognizable profile of illness as you experience it, and to help the homeopath identify the most appropriate remedies.

Choosing a remedy

You know how it hurts when you get a backache You know whether the pain localizes on one side of your back or if it travels up or down your spine. You know if it was triggered by overexertion, by rainy weather, or a flare-up of a degenerative or inflammatory illness. If you suffer from chronic backaches, you will know from the first hint of a symptom whether this one will be protracted and incapacitating or transient and tolerable. If you get backaches you know these things—and this knowledge will help you to determine an appropriate homeopathic remedy.

Review your responses to the diagnostic interview, organizing your symptoms in the same categories that are given in the Materia Medica. When you consider a remedy, you are looking for a description that matches the greatest number of your particular symptoms. It is unlikely that you will experience the full range of symptoms described, so don't discount a remedy that includes some symptoms you are not experiencing.

Comparing similar remedies

Sometimes more than one remedy seems appropriate. A careful comparison of their descriptions and your symptoms will usually reveal one or more significant defining characteristics. The following example demonstrates how to compare two similar remedies in the case of headache. The procedure is the same for any problem. If after analyzing two similar remedies, you are still unable to identify one as more suitable than the other, then just pick one and try it. If it helps, use it as long as it continues to help. If you notice no improvement within two hours, try the other.

If after analyzing your responses to the diagnostic

interview, you find that you frequently get headaches when you are under stress trying to make a deadline, list your symptoms like this:

Onset: From deadline stress.
Location: Temples. Sometimes radiates across forehead. Eyestrain. Stiff neck.
Sensation: Long slow waves of pain. Prickly pain.
Concomitants: Blurred vision (eyestrain). Nausea.
Better: Cold drinks. Keeping the window open or sitting in front of a fan.
Worse: At night.

Looking through the Materia Medica you will find that Argentum nitricum (Arg-n) and Iris versicolor (Iris) encompass symptoms of stress, blurred vision (eyestrain), nausea, better with cold, and worse at night. Both are better with cold: Arg-n with "Cold. Fresh air" (the open window and fan), Iris with "Cold drinks." Both include vomiting, which despite the nausea is not one of your symptoms. Arg-n includes trembling and a craving for sweets, which you are not experiencing. You also don't have nerve pains throughout your face and intense ringing or buzzing in your ears, which are Iris symptoms. Neither description includes stiff neck. Nevertheless, these two remedies are strong candidates and the deciding factors will be more specificity regarding location, sensation, and onset.

Location: Arg-n tends to be right-sided or frontal pain, and Iris is more commonly left-sided. Your forehead and temples (left and right side) hurt. Arg-n includes both (right side, front). Iris includes one (left side).
Sensation: Arg-n pain increases and decreases gradually (matching your "long slow waves of pain"). The "prickly" quality of the pain is a symptom that could

go either way. It suggests the nerve pain of Iris, but since it is localized in your forehead and not "over the face" it could be considered part of the Arg-n picture.

Onset: Thinking about the onset, you realize that your headaches come on while you are working, which is another characteristic of Arg-n. Iris headaches arise when the stress ends.

For a headache with this particular constellation of symptoms, Arg-n is a better overall match than Iris.

SUMMARY OF REMEDIES FOR BACKACHE TYPES

Injury

Overexertion: Strain, sprain, spasm
Aesculus hippocastanum. Agaricus muscarius. Argentum metallicum. Arnica. Belladonna. Bryonia. Calcarea carbonica. Causticum. Cimicifuga racemosa. Gelsemium. Graphites. Hypericum. Kali carbonicum. Lycopodium. Nux vomica. Phosphorus. Pulsatilla. Rhus toxicodendron. Sepia. Silica.

Impact injuries
Aesculus hippocastanum. Agaricus muscarius. Arnica. Bryonia. Hypericum. Sepia. Silica.

Fractures
Arnica. Bryonia. Eupatorium perfoliatum.

Nerve disorders

Herniated disk, Pinched nerve
Agaricus muscarius. Belladonna. Bryonia. Causticum. Colocynthis. Graphites. Hypericum. Nux vomica. Phosphorus. Pulsatilla. Rhus toxicodendron. Zinc.

Sciatica
Belladonna. Berberis vulgaris. Bryonia. Calcarea carbonica. Colocynthis. Hypericum. Kali carbonicum. Pulsatilla. Rhus toxicodendron. Sepia. Silica. Sulphur. Zinc.

   left-sided: Causticum.
   right-sided: Lycopodium.

Inflammatory illnesses

Arthritis
Aesculus hippocastanum. Agaricus muscarius. Argentum metallicum. Belladonna. Berberis vulgaris. Bryonia. Calcarea carbonica. Causticum. Colocynthis. Gelsemium. Phosphorus. Pulsatilla. Silica. Sulphur.

Rheumatism
Aesculus hippocastanum. Argentum metallicum. Belladonna. Bryonia. Causticum. Cimicifuga racemosa. Eupatorium perfoliatum. Gelsemium. Phosphorus. Pulsatilla. Rhus toxicodendron. Sepia. Silica. Sulphur. Zinc.

Fibromyalgia
Belladonna. Berberis vulgaris. Bryonia. Calcarea carbonica. Causticum. Cimicifuga racemosa. Colocynthis. Gelsemium. Kali carbonicum. Nux vomica. Phosphorus. Pulsatilla. Rhus toxicodendron. Silica. Sulphur. Zinc.

Colds and Flu
Aesculus hippocastanum. Belladonna. Bryonia. Eupatorium perfoliatum. Gelsemium. Phosphorus. Pulsatilla. Silica.

Degenerative diseases

Bone diseases, spurs
Calcarea carbonica. Lycopodium (bone degeneration) Silica.

Osteoporosis
Argentum metallicum. Calcarea carbonica. Phosphorus.

Premenstrual and menstrual backache

Berberis vulgaris. Cimicifuga racemosa. Gelsemium. Pulsatilla. Sepia.

Injuries and Nerve Disorders

	S/O	W	In	Fr	HD	Sc
Aesculus hippocastanum		•	•			
Agaricus muscarius	•		•		•	
Argentum metallicum	•					
Arnica	•	•	•	•		
Belladonna		•				
Berberis vulgaris		•	•			•
Bryonia	•	•	•	•		•
Calcarea carbonica	•	•				
Causticum	•	•			•	•
Cimicifuga racemosa	•	•				
Colocynthis					•	•
Eupatorium perfoliatum		•		•		
Gelsemium	•	•				
Graphites	•	•				
Hypericum		•	•		•	•
Kali carbonicum	•					•
Lycopodium		•				•
Nux vomica	•	•				
Phosphorus	•					
Pulsatilla	•	•				•
Rhus toxicodendron	•				•	•
Sepia	•		•			•
Silica	•	•	•			•
Sulphur		•				•
Zinc						

Injury
S/O   Strain, sprain, spasm
      Overexertion
W   Whiplash
In   Injuries
Fr   Fractures

Nerve disorders
HD   Herniated disk,
      pinched nerve
Sc   Sciatica

Inflammatory Illnesses, Degenerative Diseases, Premenstrual and Menstrual Backache

	Ar	Rh	Fb	C/F	Bd	O	Mn
Aesculus hippocastanum	•	•					
Agaricus muscarius	•						
Argentum metallicum	•	•				•	
Arnica							
Berberis vulgaris	•						•
Belladonna							
Bryonia	•						
Calcarea carbonica	•		•		•	•	
Causticum	•	•	•				
Cimicifuga racemosa		•					•
Colocynthis	•						
Eupatorium perfoliatum		•		•			
Gelsemium	•	•					
Graphites							
Hypericum							
Kali carbonicum			•				
Lycopodium					•		
Nux vomica							
Phosphorus	•				•		
Pulsatilla	•	•					•
Rhus toxicodendron		•					
Sepia		•					•
Silica	•	•			•		
Sulphur	•	•					
Zinc		•					

Inflammatory illnesses

Ar   Arthritis
Rh   Rheumatism
Fb   Fibromyalgia
C/F   Colds and Flu

Degenerative diseases

Bd   Bone diseases, spurs
O   Osteoporosis
Mn   Premenstrual and
      menstrual backache

Remedies by Area Affected

Body part	Stiffness	Weakness	Pain

Neck	Arnica
	Belladonna
	Bryonia
	Calcarea
	   carbonica
	Cimicifuga
	   racemosa
	Silica
	Sulphur
		Aesculus
		   hippocastanum
			Belladonna
			Berberis vulgaris
			Causticum
			Eupatorium
			   perfoliatum
			Gelsemium
			Graphites
			Hypericum
			Nux vomica
			Pulsatilla

Shoulders	Belladonna		Bryonia Gelsemium Graphites Hypericum Lycopodium Nux vomica Pulsatilla Rhus toxicodendron Sulphur

Shoulder blades	Causticum		Aesculus
			   hippocastanum
			Calcarea
			   carbonica
			Gelsemium
			Phosphorus
			Pulsatilla
			Sepia
			Sulphur
			Zinc

Spine		Aesculus
		   hippocastanum
		Phosphorus
		Silica
			Agaricus
			   muscarius
			Graphites
			Hypericum
			Phosphorus
			Zinc

Remedies by Area Affected

Body part	Stiffness	Weakness	Pain
Lower back	Rhus toxicodendron	Calcarea carbonica Eupatorium perfoliatum Graphites Kali carbonicum Sepia	Belladonna Berberis vulgaris Bryonia Geisemium Graphites Hypericum Kali carbonicum Lycopodium Sepia Sulphur Zinc
Hips/sacrum/coccyx			Aesculus hippocastanum Agaricus muscarius Belladonna Causticum Cimicifuga racemosa Colocynthis Gelsemium Graphites Hypericum Kali carbonicum Pulsatilla
Legs	Argentum metallicum	Aesculus hippocastanum Argentum metallicum Kali carbonicum Nux vomica Silica	Aesculus hippocastanum Arnica Belladonna Berberis vulgaris Calcarea carbonica Causticum Cimicifuga racemosa Colocynthis Gelsemium Hypericum Kali carbonicum Pulsatilla Rhus toxicodendron

MATERIA MEDICA

AESCULUS HIPPOCASTANUM
Aesc
(Horse Chestnut)

Helpful for: Lower back pain; backache affecting sacrum, hips, pelvis. Sprain, strain, spasm. Whiplash. Injury to tailbone, hips, pelvis. Arthritis. Ankylosing spondylitis. Rheumatism. Colds/Flu. Backache with weakness in any area, weakness extends to legs.

Sensation: Chilliness up and down back. Flying pains all over. Dragging pain in pelvis. Hot and dry, stiff and rough. Aching. Bruised pain, especially through the sacrum and across the hips. Lameness in neck. Aching between shoulder blades.

Modalities

Better: Cool open air. Bathing. Kneeling.

Worse: In morning after awaking. Motion, much worse walking. Standing. Stooping. Cold and cold seasons.

Concomitants: Lower bowel problems, hemorrhoids, constipation. Pain with bowel movements. Frontal head-

ache (worse in the morning). Spine feels weak. Back and legs give out. Varicose veins. Limbs aching and sore. Fullness in various parts (nose, sinuses, chest, abdomen, bowels, joints). Dryness. Swollen glands, congestion.
Mentals & Generals: Depressed, gloomy, and irritable. Distressed when not busy. Feels something is missing. Wakes up confused, bewildered.

The pain and weakness—the back just "gives out"— are so severe that the person is unable to work and walking is virtually impossible. The backache affects the sacrum and hips, the spine feels weak. The person has difficulty rising from a sitting position and may make several attempts before being successful. The backache may feel like a tearing pain in the small of the back or feel as if the back would break.

The concomitant symptom of fullness (varicosity, constipation) or a sensation of fullness is characteristic of this remedy.

AGARICUS MUSCARIUS
Agar
(Toadstool, Amanita)

Helpful for: Sprain, strain, spasm. Overexertion. Spine injury. Herniated disk. Arthritis. Ankylosing spondylitis.

Sensation: Frostbite symptoms: cold, numbness, and tingling or itching, redness, and burning. Shooting, burning pain up and down the spine, as if it were on fire. Cold spots along spine, as if pierced by needles of ice. Hypersensitive to touch. Back and neck feel dislocated. Pain in sacrum. Violent bearing-down pains. Symptoms may appear diagonally, for example, left arm and right leg.

Modalities

Better: Evening. Warmth. Moving around slowly.

Worse: Pressure. Cold or freezing air or weather. Drinking cold water. After sex. Before thunderstorms. Women may feel worse in the morning during menses.

Concomitants: Jerking, twitching, trembling, itching are strong indications. No twitching when asleep. Numbness in legs. Dull headache, especially one in which the head keeps falling backward. Heart palpitations. The skin, especially on the soles of the feet, is itchy and burning.

Mentals & Generals: Extremely talkative, talks in rhymes, incoherent speech. Conscious or unconscious singing. Lethargic during the day, but comes alive at night. Abuses alcohol and/or drugs. Moods alternate between silly, talkative, and manic and depressed and indifferent. Clumsy and awkward, drops things, bumps into things. Craves eggs, sweets, and salt. Sleeps fitfully, vivid dreaming, starts awake. Paroxysms of yawning. Dizzy from sunlight and when walking.

Agaricus people are very concerned about their health and fearful of cancer. They are hypersensitive to cold and damp environments. Twitching anywhere (facial tics, muscular twitches), twitching that ceases when the person is asleep, involuntary laughter (laughing follows yawning or pressure on the spine), and the sensation of being pierced by needles of ice are defining characteristics for this remedy.

The effects of Agaricus are similar to those of Hypericum. If the spine is extremely sensitive to pressure and touch, give Agaricus first. If there are shooting pains, give Hypericum, then follow with Agaricus if necessary. A defining distinction between the two remedies is the symptom of jerking and twitching: if it continues during sleep, give Hypericum; if it stops during sleep, give Agaricus.

ARGENTUM METALLICUM
Arg-m
(Silver)

Helpful for: Sprain, strain, spasm. Overexertion. Arthritis. Ankylosing spondylitis. Rheumatism. Hip-joint diseases. Joint disorders. Osteoporosis.

Sensation: Severe backache. Walks bent over. Icy cold feeling near sacrum. Painless twitching or electriclike shocks. Bones are very painful, tender.

Modalities

Better: In open air. Coffee. Motion. Wrapping up.

Worse: From touch. Toward noon. Cold damp. Lying on back, sitting, stooping, riding in a car.

Concomitants: Legs weak and trembling especially going up or down stairs. Rheumatic joints, especially elbow and knee. Limbs feel numb or stiff. Swollen ankles. Hoarseness, cough, dry mouth, weak chest.

Mentals & Generals: Hurried feeling, feels that time is passing slowly. Melancholy. Cries from nervous irritation. Restless anxiety. Weakness and fatigue drives the person to lie down. Great appetite, even after eating a full meal or so averse to eating that even the thought of food provokes nausea. Thirstless, even with fever. Restless sleep.

The chief action of Argentum metallicum is on the joints and their component elements: bones, cartilage, and ligaments. Typical symptoms are tearing and bruised pains, tenderness and weakness, rheumatic pain without swelling.

The remedy is especially helpful with left-sided ailments. Emaciation and dryness are also characteristic.

Arnica
Arn
(Leopard's bane, Mountain daisy)

Helpful for: Sprain, strain, spasm. Overexertion. Whiplash. Injury. Fracture.

CAUTION: Head or back injuries and headache or backache following an injury, *must* be evaluated by a medical doctor.

Sensation: A bruised, sore feeling. Sore and aching. Muscles of neck weak, head falls backward or to either side.

Modalities

Better: Lying down or with head low. Open air. Warm.

Worse: With the least touch or pressure. Motion, physical exertion. Damp cold. Hot sun.

Concomitants: Limbs ache as if beaten. Sprained and dislocated feeling. Gout.

Mentals & Generals: Wants to be left alone, fears being touched. Very fearful, like a wounded animal. Fears sickness, the approach of anyone. Fearful at night and upon waking. Gloomy. Irritable, wants to be left alone. Overworked and exhausted. May be accident-prone and/or experience a loss of confidence due to accidents. Loss of appetite during the day, but fiercely hungry at night. Severe fatigue causes restlessness and sleeplessness.

In most cases of injury, give Arnica first to remove the effects of the shock, then follow it with a remedy appropriate to the symptoms. Arnica patients tend to have a high tolerance for pain, sometimes to the point of not realizing how badly they are injured or of denying there is a problem at all. In any case where the sensation is "achy, bruised, sore all over," think of Arnica.

BELLADONNA
Bell
(Deadly nightshade)

Helpful for: Sprain, strain, spasm. Overexertion. Whiplash. Herniated disk. Sciatica. Arthritis. Rheumatism. Fibromyalgia. Cold/Flu. Nonspecific lower back pain. Stiff neck.

Sensation: Severe neuralgic pains. Throbbing, shooting, stabbing. Hot, burning. Heavy, full. Pain in nape. Stiff neck and right shoulder. The neck is so stiff, it feels as if it could break. Lower back pain with pain in hips and thighs. Pain runs from head downward.

Modalities

Better: With warm wraps. Bending head backward. Firm pressure applied gradually. Semi-erect posture. Bed rest.

Worse: Cold and drafts. Lying down. Touch. Noise. With motion: jarring, stepping, stooping, or bending head forward, rising up. Between 3 P.M. and 9 P.M.

Concomitants: Restlessness. Redness, flushed face. Dilated pupils. Rush of blood to the head. Dizziness when moving head. Blood in nasal mucous. Extremities ice cold. Congestion. Skin rashes. Eyes staring and brilliant, pupils dilated.

Mentals & Generals: Jerking and twitching. Restlessness. May rock violently back and forth. Sleepy, but cannot sleep; starts awake when falling asleep. Moans and tosses about while sleeping. Cries out or screams in sleep. Senses hyperacute. Mental excitation. Furious, quarrelsome, strikes out in a rage. Delirium, nightmares, may hallucinate. Disinclined to talk. Changeable; perversity, with tears. Loss of appetite. Desire for lemons and lemonade, which are soothing. Headache from overexposure to sun.

Belladonna's most outstanding characteristics are: sudden and intense pain; pain that comes and goes abruptly (with anxiety about the return of the pain); hot, red, shiny skin; swelling or a feeling of congestion; throbbing; hyperacuity of the senses and restlessness, especially restless sleep. The patient may have a flushed face; glassy, staring eyes; dilated pupils; and a dry mouth but no thirst. Her limbs may jerk or twitch convulsively. Belladonna is also associated with an excited mental state and with delirium, especially if there is fever. It is also useful for the acute early stages of inflammatory illnesses characterized by high fever and severe pain.

The patient may be kept awake by pain from pulsating blood vessels or the sound of heartbeats reverberating in her head. When awake, her attention is focused inward; she may seem dazed and unresponsive or speak nonsensically.

BERBERIS VULGARIS
Berb
(Barberry)

Helpful for: Whiplash. Herniated disk. Sciatica. Arthritis. Fibromyalgia. Menstrual backache. Backache with kidney or bladder infection. Postoperative pain.

Sensation: Sharp stabbing pain, as if a thorn were stuck in the back. Stitching pain in back and neck. Pain radiates from small of back. Deep pain in the lower back. Bubbling sensation in kidney area, over the skin, or in joints. Pain that moves from side to side. Shooting pain down leg.

Modalities

Better: Standing.

Worse: Left side. Motion, walking. Rising from sitting. Breathing aggravates pain. Twilight and at night.

Concomitants: Gout. Kidney or liver trouble. Enlarged prostate. Urinary trouble: burning, painful, frequent urination, incontinence. Rheumatic pain in extremities. Swollen neck glands. Intense weariness in legs after walking a short distance. Frontal headache. Pain in thighs and loins when urinating. Sweats from slightest exertion.

Mentals & Generals: Mentally and physically tired. Person finds it difficult to concentrate; the train of thought is easily disrupted. Sleepy during the day. Sleep is restless, unrefreshing with anxious dreams and frequent waking.

Berberis people are listless, apathetic, and indifferent. They have alternating contrary symptoms, for example, thirst and thirstless, hunger and no appetite, chills and fever. Berberis is helpful in conditions where pain radiates from the back and where there are many old troubles in the back.

BRYONIA
Bry
(Wild hops)

Helpful for: Sprain, strain, spasm. Overexertion. Whiplash. Injury. Fracture. Herniated disk. Sciatica. Arthritis. Ankylosing spondylitis. Rheumatism. Fibromyalgia. Colds/Flu.

Sensation: Stiffness. Fullness and heaviness. Throbbing pain on motion. Pain in shoulders. Stiff neck. Stitches and stiffness in small of back, worse walking or turning.

Modalities

Worse: Slightest motion or any exertion. From light touch. From heat, especially in a warm and stuffy room. Sitting up. Light. After eating. From coughing. In the morning. Sudden changes in weather.

Better: Stillness, especially lying still in a dark room. Firm pressure, especially on painful area. Coolness, open air. Person should avoid cold, however, as this may trigger a headache.

Concomitants: Thirsty and dry. Bitter taste in the mouth. May vomit after eating or drinking, especially after warm drinks. Hot head. Red congested eyes; sore eyeballs. Splitting headache. Nausea and faintness on rising or lifting head. May be constipated.

Mentals & Generals: Must keep perfectly still. Peevish, wants to be left alone. Dull mind, slow, sluggish, passive. May feel homesick, even if at home. Headache precedes or accompanies other illnesses. Symptoms may be worse after a meal, especially after eating vegetables.

The outstanding characteristic of Bryonia is aggravation with motion; any exertion, even moving the eyes or shifting position when sitting or lying down, will increase the pain. Bryonia is sometimes called the ''sleeping bear'' remedy. The patient prefers ''denning up:'' being left alone in a dark place and will be irritable, snappish, or possibly violent if disturbed. A second characteristic is dryness: dry mouth, possibly with cracked lips, dry nose and/or throat, dry cough (especially at night), great thirst at long intervals with a desire for large quantities.

CALCAREA CARBONICA
Calc, Calc carb
(Carbonate of lime)

Helpful for: Sprain, strain, spasm. Overexertion. Whiplash. Sciatica. Arthritis. Fibromyalgia. Bone diseases (spurs, curvature). Osteoporosis.

Sensation: As if sprained. Neck stiff and rigid, worse from lifting. Pain between shoulder blades. Back, especially the small of the back, too weak to sit upright in a chair. Vertebrae feel loose. Weakness and "sinking" sensations. Pain deep in muscles. Swollen joints.

Modalities

Worse: Change in weather. Cold in every form. Wet weather. Open air. Mental or physical exertion, worry. Standing, lifting, or stooping. Letting limbs hang down.

Better: Dry climate and weather. Lying still, lying on painful side. Rubbing, scratching, any soothing with hands.

Concomitants: Increased perspiration, night sweats. Cold hands and feet. Tearing pains or cramps in extremities. Dizziness, nausea. Face pale. Ravenous hunger and craving for indigestible things (chalk, dirt, pencils). Aversion to fats. Craves eggs. Large appetites with slow digestion.

Mentals & Generals: Overworked and exhausted. Jaded state, mentally or physically, due to overwork, assuming too much responsibility. Feel they need to do everything themselves, others "won't do it right." Generally passive, but may become obstinate, if asked to do something they don't want to do. Easy relapses, interrupted convalescence. Apprehensive toward evening, may be afraid of the dark. Forgetful or slow-witted. Insomnia, nightmares.

People who benefit most from Calcarea have a chilly constitution, the slightest cold "goes right through" them. They crave warmth. They may feel cold all the time and have trouble keeping warm. (Distinct from Sulphur conditions where the person feels overheated and seeks cold.) They may become ill after being out in the rain.

A second outstanding characteristic is localized or general perspiration which may be profuse and sour-smelling—head sweats that wet the pillow, for example. Calcarea people may have cold, clammy feet; the feeling is as if they were wearing damp socks.

CAUSTICUM
Caust
(Hahnemann's Tinctura acris sine Kali)

Helpful for: Muscle spasm. Whiplash. Herniated disk, pinched nerve. Sciatica (left-sided). Arthritis. Rheumatism. Fibromyalgia.

Sensation: Burning pain. Soreness. Rawness. Tearing pains in joints and bones, muscles and fibers. Stiff joints. Stiffness between shoulders. Pain worse when swallowing. Dull pain in nape of neck. Bruised, darting pains in coccyx. Pain goes forward or to the thighs. Cramps in lower back and buttocks. Pain in hips, worse when coughing. Paralytic weakness.

Modalities

Better: Cold drinks. Damp, wet weather. Warmth of bed. Gentle motion.

Worse: Clear, fine weather. Dry, cold air. Wind, drafts. Extremes of temperature. Stooping. 3–4 A.M. Riding in cars. Exertion.

Concomitants: Rigid tissue. Contractures. Weakness, progressive loss of muscular strength. Numbness in the extremities. Paralysis. Restless legs at night. Walks unsteadily, falls easily (weak ankles). Hemorrhoids. Sour or acid stomach. Hoarseness, coughing.

Mentals & Generals: Susceptible to ill effects from cold and heat. Hopeless, despondent, wants to die. Memory fails (mental paralysis). Apprehensive, feels conscience-stricken. Hungry, but loses appetite when food is presented. Averse to sweets. Yawning and stretching, very drowsy. Restless while sleeping—much movement of the arms and legs.

Note: Causticum was first compounded by Samuel Hahnemann. Its exact chemical composition is not documented, but it is believed to include potassium hydrate or caustic potash.

Causticum is marked by paralysis of single parts, neuralgic and rheumatic pains, restlessness, and weakness. The weakness may result from a long-standing grief or from an illness. "Sinking" sensations and emaciation are also characteristic.

CIMICIFUGA RACEMOSA
Cimic
(Black snakeroot, Black Cohosh)

Helpful for: Sprain, strain, spasm. Overexertion. Whiplash. Rheumatism. Fibromyalgia. Premenstrual and menstrual backache. Lower back pain.

Sensation: Spine, especially upper spine, very sensitive. Low back pain extends to hips and thighs. Stiffness and cramp or contraction in neck and back. Pain like electric shocks. Cramp.

Modalities

Better: Warmth. Rest. Eating.

Worse: Night and morning. Cold, damp air. Change of weather. Sitting. During menses.

Concomitants: Restless extremities. Pelvic pain, pain from hip to hip. Women have pain before menses. Rheumatic, aching pain in ribs. Limbs feel heavy and achy with muscular soreness. Feels generally sick and exhausted. Tinnitus. Headache with hypersensitivity to light and intense aching deep in eyes.

Mentals & Generals: Sleeplessness. Gloomy and dejected, feels under a dark cloud. Talkative, with frequent changing from subject to subject. Variable appetite, great thirst. Face pale, hot.

Cimicifuga is primarily a remedy for women, but it should not be overlooked by a man who experiences the kind of low back and pelvic pain described here. Cimicifuga is useful in cases of muscle cramp, and where there is trembling or shuddering, twitching or jerking limbs, and numbness or weakness.

COLOCYNTHIS
Coloc
(Bitter cucumber)

Helpful for: Herniated disk, pinched nerve. Sciatica. Arthritis. Fibromyalgia. Lower back pain.

Sensation: Cramplike pain in hip. Pain from hip to knee. Pain shoots down leg. Severe pain. Cramping, twitching, constriction, contraction. As if clamped with iron bands. As if stabbed by a spear. Pain may be burning, digging, rending, or tearing. Waves of pain. Shooting, lightning-like pain. Muscles feel contracted, too short. Stiff, painful joints.

Modalities

Better: Warmth. Firm pressure. Lying with knees drawn up to chest. Coffee.

Worse: Resting on back, from stooping, moving eyelids. Change of season. Cold winds. Damp weather.

Concomitants: Headache with nausea and vomiting. Bitter taste in mouth. Severe abdominal pain or cramping.

Mentals & Generals: Irritable, short-tempered, angry, indignant. Mortification from offense. May scream from the pain.

Colocynthis is marked by spasms and cramping, the patient will bend double and writhe with the pain. They are better with hard pressure and may lean against a chair or the wall or press something hard (like a book) against the painful area. Colocynthis is similar to Magnesia phosphorica but more severe, more left-sided, and better with hard pressure (worse heat).

People who benefit from this remedy are embittered by their pain; they want to be left alone and not bothered. They may have a deep suppressed rage or have experienced years of frustration.

EUPATORIUM PERFOLIATUM
Eup-per
(Bone-set)

Helpful for: Whiplash. Fractures. Rheumatism. Bone pain. Colds/flu.

Sensation: Aching back pain. Aching in bones with extreme soreness of flesh. Aching in arms and wrists. Gouty soreness and inflamed nodes of joints, associated with headache. Pain in back of neck and between the shoulders. Intense backache, as if beaten, pain ascends. Trembling in back during fever. Beating pain in nape and base of skull, better after rising. Aching pain in the back as if from a bruise. Weakness in small of back.

Modalities

Better: Resting on hands and knees. After vomiting. Sweating. Lying face down.

Worse: Cold air. Periodically, marked periodicity (7–9 A.M. every third or fourth day). Lying on painful part. Motion. Coughing.

Concomitants: Influenza, chills and fever. Muscles of chest, back, and limbs feel sore, achy, bruised. Throbbing headache. Pain in bones as if broken. Gout.

Mentals & Generals: Person is chilled and nauseated. Very restless, cannot keep still. Sleepiness with difficulty breathing. Stretching and yawning. At night, feels as if going out of his mind. May wake with headache. Anxious, despondent. Moans with aching pains. Thirst precedes chill. Great thirst for cold water, drinks in large drafts although drinking provokes vomiting. Sight or smell of food is nauseating.

This remedy's primary characteristic is violent aching, extreme soreness, bone-breaking pain. Also, any symptoms that are relieved by resting on the hands and knees (cough, headache, backache) suggest Eup-per.

GELSEMIUM
Gels
(Yellow Jasmine)

Helpful for: Sprain, strain, spasm. Overexertion. Whiplash. Arthritis. Rheumatism. Fibromyalgia. Cold/Flu. Premenstrual or menstrual backache.

Sensation: Dull, heavy, aching pain in muscles or bone. Pain runs up the back, toward the head. Chilliness up and down back. General prostration. Slightest exertion is exhausting. Muscles of neck and shoulders achy and sore. Pain under shoulder blades. Deep-seated pain in lower back, generally passes upward, but may extend to hips and legs.

Modalities

Better: Lying propped up by pillows and quite still. Pressure. Sweating; after urination. With stimulants. Fresh air.

Worse: Damp weather, fog, before a storm (falling barometer). Emotion or excitement (especially bad news). In midmorning (10 A.M.). Mental effort, heat of sun, tobacco smoke.

Concomitants: Great weakness and trembling of the limbs. Tottering gait. Dizziness, originating at base of skull. Nausea.

Mentals & Generals: The outstanding symptom for Gelsemium is extreme fatigue and sleepiness, the patient simply *cannot* stay awake. If awake, the patient is groggy and lethargic. Very dull-witted, can't rally enough energy to think. The slightest exertion is profoundly exhausting.

Gelsemium differs from Bryonia in the absolute quality of the exhaustion. Bryonia patients are irritable if disturbed, a Gelsemium patient is too tired to be irritable, too tired to sleep, too tired to eat or drink anything.

Gelsemium is especially helpful for viral infections and for elderly people who are susceptible to infections and who are, or believe that they are, frail.

GRAPHITES
Graph
(Black lead, Plumbago)

Helpful for: Sprain, strain, spasm. Overexertion. Whiplash. Herniated disk. Spinal pain. Neck pain. Lower back pain.

Sensation: Spinal pains. Pain in small of back with great weakness. Pain in nape of neck and shoulders,. Sacral pains with crawling. Numbness of sacrum, down the legs. Pain in lumbar region as if vertebrae were broken.

Modalities

Better: After walking in open air.

Worse: Looking up or stooping the head. Cold and drafts. Motion. When hungry. Warmth of bed.

Concomitants: Limbs are burning, cramping, jerking. Arms and legs go to sleep. Legs swell. Toes stiff and contracted. Eczema. Burning in old scars. Old scars ulcerate.

Mentals & Generals: Sad, fearful, irresolute, hesitates at trifles. Unable to decide. Feels miserable and unhappy. Weeps without cause, or when listening to music. Impulse to groan. Fidgety while sitting at work. Sleepless until midnight. Does not feel refreshed in the morning. Averse to meat, fish, cooked food. Sweets provoke nausea.

Graphites is indicated in people whose senses are hyperacute and who take cold easily. They cannot tolerate the smell of flowers, for example, or prefer to rest in the dark. Their breathing may be affected with a sensation of suffocation that wakes them at night. There may be muscle spasms and twitching, especially of the limbs or eyelids. An outstanding characteristic of Graphites is skin eruptions—old scars that ooze, weeping eczema, ulceration—or skin that is rough and dry and breaks easily.

HYPERICUM
Hyper
(St. John's wort)

Helpful for: Spasms after an injury. Whiplash. Injuries, especially from falling or from a blow. Herniated disk, pinched nerve. Sciatica. Tailbone pain.

Sensation: Painfully sensitive spine. Pain in nape of neck. Cervical vertebrae very sensitive to touch. Lower back pain. Pressure over sacrum. Violent pain and inability to walk after injury to coccyx. Shooting pain from injured spot. Tearing, rheumatic, shaking pains. Tingling, burning, numbness. Paralytic weakness. Prickling, as from being stuck with needles. Shuddering. Joints feel bruised.

Modalities

Better: Lying face down. Bending head back.

Worse: Shock. Exertion. Jarring. Light touch. Change of weather, fog, cold, damp.

Concomitants: Headache. Darting pains in shoulders. Crawling sensations in hands and feet. Jerks, sharp pains in the limbs. Limbs feel detached.

Mentals & Generals: Nervous depression, especially after an accident. Melancholy. Irritable. Weak memory. Makes mistakes in writing, forgets what she wanted to say. Feels lifted high in the air, or has anxiety about falling from a great height. Appetite increases in morning and evening. Great thirst. Drowsy. Talks wildly in sleep, especially after 4 A.M. Limbs jerk and twitch while sleeping (distinct from Agaricus muscarius, where spasms cease during sleep). Vertigo.

The outstanding characteristics of Hypericum are radiating pain, shooting pain, and very sensitive to touch. Hypericum is especially suited for injuries to areas that are rich in nerve endings (fingertips, the spine, the coccyx). It also aids the healing of puncture wounds and lacerations.

The effects of Hypericum are similar to those of Agaricus muscarius. A defining distinction between the two remedies is the symptom of jerking and twitching. If it continues during sleep, give Hypericum. If it stops during sleep, give Agaricus. Also, if the primary symptom is that the spine is extremely sensitive to pressure and touch, give Agaricus first. If there are shooting pains, however, start with Hypericum and follow with Agaricus if necessary.

Note: Homeopathic Hypericum can be used to relieve the mental and emotional consequences of injury—fright, anxiety, and the effects of shock. However, it is not recommended for the categories of depression that respond to herbal preparations of St. John's wort.

KALI CARBONICUM
Kali c
(Carbonate of Potassium)

Helpful for: Sprain, strain, spasm. Overexertion. Sciatica. Fibromyalgia. Lower back pain.

CAUTION: Do not use if fever is present.

Sensation: Back feels as if broken. Stiffness and paralytic pain in back. Burning in spine. Severe backache during pregnancy. Lower back feels weak. Back and legs give out. Lumbago with sudden sharp pains extending up and down. Stitching pain in kidney region. Hip disease. Pain in buttocks, hip joints, thighs. Pains are sharp and cutting. Stitching pain. Throbbing pain.

Modalities

Better: Motion. Warm humid weather. Open air. Sitting with elbows on knees.

Worse: Cold air in cold weather. Drafts. Early morning. Sudden or unguarded motion.

Concomitants: Joints give way. Tearing pains in limbs. Pain from hip to knee. Soles of feet very sensitive, limbs jerk if feet are lightly touched. Violent "sick" headache. Oppression of breathing.

Mentals & Generals: Person feels compelled to lie down or lean against something. Peevish, irritable, quarrelsome, weepy. Anxious. Hypersensitive to pain, noise, touch. Never wants to be left alone. Alternating moods. Desire for sweets and acids. Milk and warm food disagree. Hunger exacerbates emotional and physical condition. Drowsy after eating. Talks in sleep. Awakes between 1 A.M. and 4 A.M., cannot get to sleep again.

Sweat, backache, and weakness are the defining characteristics of Kali carbonicum. The "touchiness" of the remedy, both physically and emotionally, is also marked.

The person is easily startled by any sound or by light touch. The remedy is more right-sided than left. It is helpful for people who take cold easily.

LYCOPODIUM
Lyc
(Club moss)

Helpful for: Sprain, strain, spasm. Overexertion. Whiplash. Sciatica (right side). Degenerative bone disease.

Sensation: Burning between shoulder blades, like hot coals. Lower back pain. Stiff back. Emaciation around neck. Bubbling sensations. Numbness. Tearing pains in shoulder and elbow joints. Twitching and jerking.

Modalities

Better: Motion, especially restlessness better with motion. Warm drinks. Cool air. From uncovering, especially uncovering the head.

Worse: Between 4–8 P.M. Cold food or drink. Sitting erect.

Concomitants: Bones ache at night. Shakes head without apparent cause. Facial contortions. Hands and feet numb; limbs go to sleep. Right foot hot, left cold. Gout. Gassy, constipation or diarrhea.

Mentals & Generals: Nervous excitement and prostration. Wants to be alone, but wants to know that someone is nearby if needed. Cranky on waking; may wake from hunger. Bullying tendency, with bluff and bravado. Fear of failure, of breaking down under stress. Great hunger easily satisfied or arising soon after a large meal. Craves sweets, warm food and drink.

Lycopodium patients attempt to cover an inner sense of inadequacy by putting up fronts, by pretending to be something they're not. An analogy is made with the Cowardly Lion in *The Wizard of Oz,* who hid an inner timidity beneath a mask of bluff and bluster. Lycopodium people tend to be overdeveloped mentally—they believe it is safer to think than to feel.

NUX VOMICA
Nux-v
(Poison-nut)

Helpful for: Sprain, strain, spasm. Overexertion. Whiplash. Herniated disk, pinched nerve. Fibromyalgia. Lower back pain.

Note: Nux is said to act best if given in the evening.

Sensation: Piercing, sticking, tearing, burning, stinging pains. Twitching or spasms. Burning in spine. Nerve pain through neck and shoulders. Sensation of sudden loss of power in arms and legs in morning. Low back pain is aggravated by turning over in bed, the person may sit up in order to turn over without pain. Backache worse lying down, must get up and walk.

Modalities

Better: Rest. In the evening. Wet weather. After a bowel movement. With heat (except wants head cool). If allowed to nap undisturbed.

Worse: Much worse in the morning, especially 3 to 4 A.M. Lying down, must get up and walk. Mental exertion. Cold, especially cold dry air. Eating, especially overeating. Stimulants. Anger.

Concomitants: Arms and hands go to sleep. Legs go numb, knees crack while walking. Headache, nausea. Very sensitive to cold, the slightest draft or coolness aggravates symptoms. Perspires freely.

Mentals & Generals: "Type A" personality: driven, given to excesses (overeats, substance abuse, especially stimulants and alcohol). Impatient, irritable, argumentative, oversensitive, touchy. Difficulty sleeping due to overactive mind or sensitivity to slight noises. Cannot sleep after 3 A.M., stays awake until morning, then may doze.

Typically, a Nux patient is thin, spare, quick, active, nervous, and irritable. He works with his mind—a student or office worker who has mental strains, cares, and anxieties and leads a sedentary life. To compensate he will seek out stimulants, such as coffee, or overindulge in sedatives, such as rich foods and alcohol or, in extreme cases, narcotics. Late hours and fitful sleep are a consequence; a thick head, indigestion, and an irritable temper follow in the morning. He may develop a dependency on cathartics to relieve constipation, antacids to soothe a chronically queasy stomach, and/or analgesics for the headache.

Nux patients are easily chilled and avoid drafts and open air. They are very irritable, fault-finding, and quarrelsome, and do not like to be touched. Their symptoms are always much worse in the morning and are aggravated by mental exertion, tobacco, alcohol, coffee, open air.

PHOSPHORUS
Phos
(Phosphorus)

Helpful for: Sprain, strain, spasm. Overexertion. Herniated disk, pinched nerve. Arthritis. Rheumatism. Fibromyalgia. Cold/Flu. Degenerative bone disease. Osteoporosis.

Sensation: Burning in back. Back pains feel as if broken, impeding all motion. Cramp, burning between shoulder blades. Weak spine. Stitching pain from coccyx to base of skull. Joints stiff with little pain, easily dislocated. Weak spells in joints.

Modalities

Better: Cold food, air, and applications. Massage, rubbing. Sitting. Lying on right side. In the dark.

Worse: Change of weather. Windy, stormy weather. Physical or mental exertion. Lying on left side, painful side, or back. Exertion.

Concomitants: Bleeding, hemorrhages. Totters while walking.

Mentals & Generals: Excitable, impressionable. Fearful, as if something were creeping out of every corner. Fears thunderstorms, being alone at twilight. Timid and irresolute. Apathetic. Wants sympathy. Craves cold, iced drinks. Craves chocolate. Ravenous hunger, hunger after eating, night eating. Catnaps. Sleepless before midnight. Sleepwalking. Vivid dreams.

Problems that respond to Phosphorus have an insidious onset, with gradually increasing debility, and ending with severe or rapid disease. Defining characteristics are burning sensations—burning in spots along the spine, between the shoulder blades—or of heat running up the spine and extreme restlessness. The person cannot stay still.

PULSATILLA
Puls
(Wind flower)

Helpful for: Sprain, strain, spasm. Overexertion. Whiplash. Herniated disk. Sciatica. Arthritis. Rheumatism. Fibromyalgia. Cold/Flu. Premenstrual and menstrual backache. Pain that extends to hips.

Sensation: Shooting pain in the nape and back, between shoulders. Pain in sacrum from sitting. Wandering, stitching pains. May be worse on the right side. Pressure, distention, throbbing. Constricting, congestive. Back feels bandaged.

Modalities

Better: Consolation. Breezes. Cold fresh air and cold applications (especially for arthritis and joint pain). Cold food and drink, though not thirsty. Walking or slow motion in open air. Pressure on painful side. Erect posture. Lying with head high. Onset of menses.

Worse: Evening, especially at twilight, and night. Heat. Pressure on painless side. Lying or sitting quiet. Motion of eyes, stooping. Wet weather.

Concomitants: Legs painful, feel heavy and weary (worse when limbs hang down). Pain in hip joint. Joints swollen and red. Pain in limbs shifts rapidly, alternates from side to side, may let up with a "snap." Menstrual or premenstrual headache. Eyes itch, profuse burning tears or bland yellowish discharge. Sour food causes vomiting.

Mentals & Generals: Weepy, clinging. Moody and changeable. Feels lonely and helpless. Craves company and sympathy and likes being fussed over. Feels better after being served "treat" foods—sweets, butter, creamy foods—that suggest affection and caring. Thirstless.

Insomnia. Sleeps in the afternoon, may sleep with hands over the head. Sleeps under blankets with a window open.

The person's disposition and mental state are the deciding factors for the use of this remedy. Pulsatilla is most effective for people with mild, gentle, yielding natures. People who are sentimental and easily moved to tears, whose moods shift "like the wind." Often they will feel better, whatever their ailment, in the open air, especially if there is a light breeze. They like to rest with their heads propped up and are uncomfortable with only one pillow. They may suffer anxiety or fears at night; primarily, they fear being alone. They are easily discouraged, crave company and sympathy, and enjoy being fussed over.

Pulsatilla and Silica are similar in their actions. Conditions appropriate for Pulsatilla are more transient—less constant, deeper-seated, or long-lived. If you are unsure of which to choose, give Pulsatilla first; if relief is incomplete, follow with Silica.

RHUS TOXICODENDRON
Rhus tox
(Poison ivy, Poison oak)

Helpful for: Sprain, strain, spasm. Overexertion. Herniated disk, pinched nerve. Sciatica. Rheumatism. Fibromyalgia. Lower back pain. Stiff neck.

Sensation: Stiffness. Pain. Rheumatic pain (hot, painful swelling of joints). Tearing pain in tendons, ligaments. Bones ache. Sciatic pain, radiates from lower back and tears down the thighs. Pain between shoulders when swallowing.

Modalities

Better: Continuous motion, walking, change of position, from stretching out limbs. Warm dry weather. Lying on something hard. Rubbing affected area.

Worse: Cold, wet, rainy weather and after rain in any season. During and after sleep or resting. At night. While sitting. Lying on back or right side.

Concomitants: Tingling or loss of sensation in feet or fingertips. Numbness, paralysis. Trembling after exertion. Itching, skin or scalp. Headache in base of skull, or one that begins in the forehead and creeps back.

Mentals & Generals: Sad and listless. Irritable. Great apprehensiveness at night, cannot remain in bed. No appetite. Craves cold drinks, although they aggravate the chill. Desire for milk. Drowsy after eating. Great restlessness, cannot remain in bed. Sleepless before midnight. Frequent violent yawning. Heavy stuporous sleep. Dreams of great exertion. Awakens tired, stiff, or sore.

Rhus tox is known as the ''rusty hinge'' remedy; its defining characteristic is pain and stiffness that are relieved by motion. (Distinct from Bryonia, which is much worse with motion.) It has marked beneficial effect on joints and tendons, nerves, and the spinal cord. It can be helpful for backache during flu.

SEPIA
Sep
(Inky juice of cuttlefish)

Helpful for: Spasms. Injury. Sciatica. Rheumatism. Premenstrual and menstrual backache. Lower back pain.

Sensation: Weak, empty, hollow feeling in lower back. Aching between shoulder blades or in lower back. Icy coldness between shoulder blades. Sudden pain, as if struck with a hammer. A "bearing down" pain in the lower back which may hinder breathing.

Modalities

Better: Vigorous motion, exercise, dancing. With legs crossed. Pressing back against something hard. Warmth. Cold drinks, cold bathing. Open air.

Worse: Cold air, snowy air, dampness, before thunderstorms.

Concomitants: Sudden prostration. Shuddering from the pain. Short walk fatigues much. Muscles jerk. Burning sensations in different parts of the body. Feels cold, even in a warm room. Stiffness. Restless limbs, twitching and jerking night and day. Coldness in legs.

Mentals & Generals: Angry, sensitive, irritable, sulky. Averse to company or sympathy, yet dreads being alone. Voracious appetite or no appetite. Sudden cravings and sudden satiety. Everything tastes too salty. Desires chocolate and acids (vinegar, pickles, lemons), though acids aggravate. Wakes frequently as if having been called.

Symptoms tend to travel upward. Weakness, coldness, and "emptiness" are defining characteristics. The person may also experience the sensation of a "ball" lodged or rolling around inside or complain of a prickling sensation like a mouse scampering around within.

SILICA
Sil
(Pure flint)

Helpful for: Sprain, strain, spasm. Overexertion. Whiplash. Injury. Sciatica. Arthritis. Rheumatism. Fibromyalgia. Cold/Flu. Bone disease (degenerative bone disease, spurs).

Sensation: Pain runs up the back, toward the head. Stiff neck with headache. Burning. Spinal irritation. Weakness, sensitive to drafts on back. Curvature.

Modalities

Better: Any warmth. Humid weather.

Worse: Change of weather. Cold air, drafts, damp. Physical or mental exertion, excitement. Touch. Pressure. Riding in car. After eating.

Concomitants: Limbs weak, cramping, feel paralyzed. Hands tremble when trying to do something. Feet icy cold and sweaty. Stitches in chest through the back. Painless throbbing in sternum. Headache while fasting.

Mentals & Generals: Obsessed with fixed ideas, for example, may focus on pins, and need to buy them, count them, store them in a special place, take them out, count them again. Great sensitivity to taking cold, overdresses for warmth. Easily fatigued. Loss of self-confidence. Fainthearted, anxious. Cries easily. Lack of appetite, excessive thirst. Averse to cooked food, especially meats. Intolerant of alcohol. Restless sleep with nightmares and frequent starting. Talks in sleep, may sleepwalk.

Silica and Pulsatilla are similar in their actions. Conditions appropriate for Silica are more constant, deeper-seated, and last longer. If you are unsure of which to choose, give Pulsatilla first, if relief is incomplete, follow with Silica.

Silica's sensitivity is a defining characteristic. It may

be physical, as the sensitivity to cold, or emotional, crying when spoken to kindly, for example. People who benefit from Silica may be sensitive to the moon's phases; their symptoms may be worse during the new and full moons.

SULPHUR
Sulph
(Sublimated sulphur)

Helpful for: Sciatica. Arthritis. Ankylosing spondylitis. Rheumatism. Fibromyalgia. Whiplash. Upper back pain: neck and shoulders. Lower back pain.

Sensation: As if vertebrae glided over one another. Drawing pain between shoulders. Stiffness, especially stiff neck. Curvature of spine. Lower back pain extends to stomach. Joints stiff and swollen. Unsteady gait. Cannot walk erect, walks stoop-shouldered, can straighten up only after moving. Inertia and feebleness of tone.

Modalities

Better: Dry, warm weather. Warm room and applications. Hot drinks. Lying on right side.

Worse: Warmth of bed. Washing or bathing. Periodically, at noon and midnight. Periodic, every 7 days. Standing. Stooping, jarring, motion.

Concomitants: Itching, worse with heat. Skin is very sensitive, may avoid washing. Top of head feels hot. Burning in palms of hands and soles of feet. Knees and ankles stiff. Hands trembling, sweaty. Migraine or migrainelike headache. Nausea and vomiting of bile. Marked congestion. Nose is dry and congested. Red, engorged face. Red eyes with tearing.

Mentals & Generals: Catnaps, rather than sleeping. Wakes at the slightest sound. Feels dull and stupid. Forgetful. Childish peevishness in adults. Selfish, no regard for others. Irritable, depressed, thin and weak (even with good appetite). Weak, faint, and hungry at 11 A.M. Desires sweets or salt, but eating them aggravates the condition and may provoke nausea or vomiting.

Sulphur conditions are red, itchy, and burning. They have a volcanic quality—they may lie dormant for long periods, then erupt suddenly and violently. Any discharges, including breath or sweat, may have an offensive odor. The kinds of ailments that respond to sulphur exhibit symptoms of burning, redness, and sudden onsets—"eruptions" that may be literal, as in the sense of skin eruptions, or figurative in the suddenness of the appearance and disappearance of the symptoms. A common symptom is itching that is worse with warmth—especially the warmth of a bed at night—and aggravated by scratching (which may cause burning). Sulphur is useful for acute conditions and complaints that relapse.

ZINCUM METALLICUM
Zinc
(Zinc)

Helpful for: Herniated disk, pinched nerve. Sciatica. Rheumatism. Fibromyalgia. Spinal disorders.

Sensation: Pain in small of back. Cannot bear to have back touched. Tension and stinging between shoulders. Tearing in shoulder blades. Spinal irritation. Dull aching in spine, worse sitting. Burning along spine.

Modalities

Better: Hard pressure. Warm open air. Motion. While eating. Rubbing or scratching.

Worse: Wine. Physical or mental exertion. Noise. Touch.

Concomitants: Stumbling, spastic gait. Totters while walking. Lameness, weakness. Trembling and twitching of various muscles. Feet in continuous motion, cannot keep still. Soles of feet sensitive. Feet and legs feel as if bugs were crawling over them. Anemia. Eczema.

Mentals & Generals: Lethargic. Defective vitality, tissues are worn out faster than they can be repaired. Weak memory. Very sensitive to noise. Muddled, stupid, repeats everything said to her. Melancholy. Averse to work, to talk. Cries out during sleep; wakes frightened, staring. Feet in motion during sleep. Sleepwalking.

The defining characteristics of zinc are fatigue (mental or physical), trembling, twitching, and fidgety feet. The restless feet are especially significant. The feet are in constant motion regardless of whether the person is awake or asleep.

Remedy Charts

Remedy	Helpful for	Sensation	Modalities	Concomitants	Mentals & Generals
Aesculus hippocastanum	Lower back: sacrum, hips, pelvis. Pain may extend to legs. Arthritis. Ankylosing spondylitis. Rheumatism. Injury to pelvis, hips, tailbone.	Chilliness up and down back. Flying pains all over. Aching, bruised pain. Weakness, back and legs give out. Pain with bowel movements. Dragging pain in pelvis.	*Better:* Cool open air. Bathing. Kneeling. *Worse:* In morning after awaking. Motion, much worse walking. Standing. Cold, cold seasons.	Lameness in neck. Aching between shoulder blades. Weakness, back and legs give out. Limbs aching and sore.	Depressed, gloomy, and irritable. Distressed when not busy. Feels something is missing. Wakes up confused, bewildered.

Remedy	Helpful for	Sensation	Modalities	Concomitants	Mentals & Generals
Agaricus muscarius	Arthritis. Ankylosing spondylitis. Spine injury. Herniated disk. Pain in sacrum. Overexertion.	Cold, numbness, and tingling or itching, redness, and burning. Shooting pain, cold spots up and down the spine. Hypersensitive to touch. Symptoms may appear diagonally, for example, left arm and right leg.	*Better:* Evening. Warmth. Moving around slowly. *Worse:* Pressure. Cold air or weather. Drinking cold water. After sex. Before thunderstorms. Women may feel worse in the morning during menses.	Jerking, twitching, trembling, itching. No twitching when asleep. Numbness in legs. Dull headache, especially one in which the head keeps falling backward. The skin, especially on the soles of the feet, is itchy and burning.	Moods alternate between silly, talkative, and manic and depressed and indifferent. Lethargic during the day, but comes alive at night. Abuses alcohol and/or drugs. Clumsy, awkward. Crave eggs, sweets, and salt. Sleeps fitfully, vivid dreaming, starts awake.

Remedy	Helpful for	Sensation	Modalities	Concomitants	Mentals & Generals
Argentum metallicum	Arthritis. Ankylosing spondylitis. Rheumatism. Hip-joint diseases. Joint disorders. Osteoporosis. Muscle cramps and spasm.	Severe backache. Walks bent over. Icy cold feeling near sacrum. Painless twitching or electriclike shocks. Bones are very painful, tender.	*Better:* In open air. Coffee. Motion. Wrapping up. *Worse:* From touch. Toward noon. Cold damp. Lying on back, sitting, stooping, riding in a car.	Legs weak and trembling especially going up or down stairs. Rheumatic joints, especially elbow and knee. Limbs feel numb or stiff. Swollen ankles. Hoarseness, cough, dry mouth, weak chest.	Hurried, feels that time is passing slowly. Melancholy. Cries from nervous irritation. Weakness and fatigue drives the person to lie down. Restless sleep. Great appetite or averse to eating. Thirstless.

Remedy	Helpful for	Sensation	Modalities	Concomitants	Mentals & Generals
Arnica	Trauma, injuries, falls, blows, contusions. Fractures. Sprains. Overexertion.	A bruised, sore feeling. Sore and aching. Muscles of neck weak, head falls backward or to either side.	*Better:* Lying down or with head low. Open air. Warm. *Worse:* With the least touch or pressure. Motion, physical exertion. Damp cold. Hot sun.	Limbs ache as if beaten. Sprained and dislocated feeling. Gout.	Very fearful, like a wounded animal. Wants to be left alone, fears being touched. Gloomy. Irritable. Loss of appetite during the day, but fiercely hungry at night. Severe fatigue causes restlessness and sleeplessness.

Remedy	Helpful for	Sensation	Modalities	Concomitants	Mentals & Generals
Belladonna	Lower back pain. Stiff neck.	Severe neuralgic pains. Throbbing, shooting, stabbing. Hot, burning. Heavy, full. Pain in nape. Stiff neck and right shoulder. The neck is so stiff, it feels like it could break. Lower back pain with pain in hips and thighs. Pain runs from head downwards.	*Better:* Bed rest. Warm wraps. Bending head backwards. Firm pressure applied gradually. Semi-erect posture. *Worse:* Cold and drafts. Lying down. Touch. Noise. Motion: jarring, stepping, stooping, or bending head forward, rising up. Between 3 P.M. and 9 P.M.	Jerking and twitching. Redness, flushed face. Dilated pupils. Dizziness when moving head. Extremities ice-cold. Congestion. Skin rashes. Eyes staring and brilliant, pupils dilated. Headache from overexposure to sun.	Restless. Sleepy, but cannot sleep. Moans, cries out or screams in sleep. Mental excitation. Senses hyperacute. Furious, quarrelsome. Disinclined to talk. Changeable; perversity, with tears. Loss of appetite. Desire for, and soothed by, lemons.

Remedy	Helpful for	Sensation	Modalities	Concomitants	Mentals & Generals
Berberis vulgaris	Arthritis. Sciatica. Menstrual backache. Backache with kidney or bladder infection. Postoperative pain.	Sharp stabbing pain, as if a thorn were stuck in the back. Stitching pain in back and neck. Pain radiates from small of back. Deep pain in the lower back. Bubbling sensation in kidney area, over the skin, or in joints. Pain that moves from side to side. Shooting pain down leg.	*Better:* Standing. *Worse:* Left side. Motion, walking. Rising from sitting. Breathing aggravates pain. Twilight and at night.	Rheumatic pain in extremities. Swollen neck glands. Intense weariness in legs after walking a short distance. Pain in thighs and loins when urinating. Urination: burning, painful, frequent, incontinence. Sweats from slightest exertion. Gout. Kidney or liver trouble.	Mentally and physically tired. Person finds it difficult to concentrate; the train of thought is easily disrupted. Sleepy during the day. Sleep is restless, unrefreshing with anxious dreams and frequent waking.

Remedy	Helpful for	Sensation	Modalities	Concomitants	Mentals & Generals
Bryonia	Arthritis. Ankylosing spondylitis. Herniated disk. Sciatica. Fractures and joint injuries. Overlifting, concussion.	Stiffness. Fullness and heaviness. Throbbing pain on motion. Pain in shoulders. Stiff neck. Stitches and stiffness in small of back, worse when walking or turning.	*Better:* Stillness, especially lying still in a dark room. Firm pressure. Coolness, open air. *Worse:* Slightest motion or exertion. In the morning. Heat, stuffy room. Sitting up. Change of weather.	Thirsty and dry. Bitter taste in the mouth. May vomit after eating or drinking, especially after warm drinks. Hot head. Splitting headache. Nausea and faintness on rising or lifting head. May be constipated.	Must keep perfectly still. Peevish, wants to be left alone. Dull mind, slow, sluggish, passive. May feel homesick, even if at home. Headache precedes or accompanies other illnesses.

Remedy	Helpful for	Sensation	Modalities	Concomitants	Mentals & Generals
Calcarea carbonica	Arthritis. Osteoporosis. Bone diseases. Bone spurs. Sciatica. Fibromyalgia. Strain, sprain and spasm. Overexertion.	As if sprained. Neck stiff and rigid, worse from lifting. Pain between shoulder blades. Back, especially the small of the back, too weak to sit upright in a chair. Vertebrae feel loose. Weakness and "sinking" sensations.	*Better:* Dry climate and weather. Lying still, lying on painful side. Rubbing, scratching. *Worse:* Cold in every form. Wet weather. Change in weather. Open air. Any exertion. Letting limbs hang down.	Increased perspiration, night sweats. Cold hands and feet. Tearing pains or cramps in extremities. Dizziness, nausea. Face pale.	Overworked and exhausted, assumes too much responsibility. Easy relapses, interrupted convalescence. Insomnia, nightmares. Great hunger; craves indigestible things (dirt, chalk). Averse to fats. Craves eggs.

Remedy	Helpful for	Sensation	Modalities	Concomitants	Mentals & Generals
Causticum	Arthritis. Rheumatism. Sciatica (left-sided). Pinched nerve. Herniated disk. Muscle spasm. Fibromyalgia.	Burning. Soreness. Rawness. Tearing pains. Paralytic weakness. Stiffness. Dull pain in nape of neck. Bruised, darting pains in coccyx. Pain goes forward or to the thighs. Cramps in lower back and buttocks. Pain in hips, worse coughing.	*Better:* Cold drinks. Damp, wet weather. Warmth of bed. Gentle motion. *Worse:* Clear, fine weather. Dry, cold air. Wind, drafts. Extremes of temperature. Stooping. 3–4 A.M. Riding in cars. Exertion.	Rigid tissue. Contractures. Weakness. Numbness in the extremities. Paralysis. Restless legs at night. Walks unsteadily, falls easily (weak ankles). Hemorrhoids. Sour or acid stomach. Hoarseness, coughing.	Susceptible to ill effects from cold and heat. Hopeless, despondent, wants to die. Memory fails (mental paralysis). Conscience-stricken. Hungry, but loses appetite when food is presented. Averse to sweets. Yawning and stretching, very drowsy. Restless while sleeping.

Remedy	Helpful for	Sensation	Modalities	Concomitants	Mentals & Generals
Cimicifuga racemosa	Lower back pain. Rheumatism. Overexertion. Premenstrual and menstrual backache.	Spine, especially upper spine, very sensitive. Lower back pain extends to hips and thighs. Stiffness and cramp or contraction in neck and back. Pain like electric shocks. Cramp.	*Better:* Warmth. Rest. Eating. *Worse:* Night and morning. Cold, damp air. Change of weather. Sitting. During menses.	Restless extremities. Pelvic pain, pain from hip to hip. Rheumatic, aching pain in ribs. Limbs feel heavy and achy with muscular soreness. Feels generally sick and exhausted.	Sleeplessness. Gloomy and dejected, feels under a dark cloud. Talkative, with frequent changing from subject to subject. Variable appetite, great thirst. Face pale, hot.

Remedy	Helpful for	Sensation	Modalities	Concomitants	Mentals & Generals
Colocynthis	Lower back pain. Arthritis. Herniated disk. Pinched nerve. Sciatica.	Severe pain: shooting, lightning-like, cramping, burning, digging, rending, or tearing. Waves of pain. As if stabbed by a spear clamped with iron bands. Stiff, painful joints. Muscles feel contracted, short.	*Better:* Warmth. Firm pressure. Lying with knees drawn up to chest. Coffee. *Worse:* Resting on back, from stooping, moving eyelids. Change of season. Cold winds. Damp weather.	Cramplike pain in hip, shoots down leg, from hip to knee. Headache with nausea and vomiting. Bitter taste in mouth. Severe abdominal pain or cramping. May scream from the pain.	Angry, irritable, short-tempered, indignant. Mortification from offense.

Remedy	Helpful for	Sensation	Modalities	Concomitants	Mentals & Generals
Eupatorium perfoliatum	Fractures. Rheumatism. Bone pain. Backache with flu or fever.	Intense aching backache, as if beaten; pain ascends. Weakness in small of back, trembling during fever. Aching in bones with extreme soreness of flesh. Pain in back of neck and between the shoulders.	*Better:* Resting on hands and knees. After vomiting. Sweating. Lying face down. *Worse:* Cold air. Periodically, marked periodicity (7–9 A.M. every third or fourth day). Lying on painful part. Mortion. Coughing.	Influenza, chills and fever. Muscles of chest, back, and limbs feel sore, achy, bruised. Throbbing headache. Pain in bones as if broken. Gout.	Person is chilled and nauseated. Very restless, cannot keep still. Sleepy, with difficulty breathing. Stretching and yawning. At night, feels as if going out of his mind. Great thirst for cold water, drinks in large drafts although drinking provokes vomiting. Sight or smell of food is nauseating.

Remedy	Helpful for	Sensation	Modalities	Concomitants	Mentals & Generals
Gelsemium	Arthritis. Muscle pain. Rheumatism. Spasms. Backache with flu or fever.	Dull, heavy, aching pain in muscles or bone. Pain runs up, toward the head. Chilliness up and down back. Muscles of neck and shoulders achy and sore. Pain under shoulder blades. Deep-seated pain in lower back, may extend to hips and legs.	*Better:* Lying propped up by pillows and quite still. Pressure. With stimulants. Fresh air. *Worse:* Damp weather, fog, before a storm. Emotion or excitement. Mid-morning (10 A.M.). Mental effort, heat of sun, tobacco smoke.	General prostration. Slightest exertion is exhausting. Great weakness and trembling of the limbs. Tottering gait. Dizziness, originating at base of skull. Nausea.	Extreme fatigue and sleepiness, the patient simply *cannot* stay awake. If awake, the patient is groggy and lethargic. Very dull-witted, can't rally enough energy to think. The slightest exertion is profoundly exhausting.

Remedy	Helpful for	Sensation	Modalities	Concomitants	Mentals & Generals
Graphites	Spinal pain. Neck pain. Lower back pain. Muscle spasms. Contractures. Overexertion.	Spinal pains. Pain in small of back with great weakness. Pain in nape of neck and shoulders. Sacral pains with crawling. Numbness of sacrum, down the legs. Pain in lumbar region as if vertebrae were broken.	*Better:* After walking in open air. *Worse:* Looking up or stooping the head. Cold and drafts. Motion. When hungry. Warmth of bed.	Limbs are burning, cramping, jerking. Arms and legs go to sleep. Legs swell. Toes stiff and contracted. Burning in old scars. Old scars ulcerate. Eczema.	Miserable, sad and tearful. Music provokes weeping. Fearful. Irresolute, hesitant at trifles. Sleepless until midnight; wakes unrefreshed. Averse to meat, fish, cooked food. Sweets provoke nausea.

Remedy	Helpful for	Sensation	Modalities	Concomitants	Mentals & Generals
Hypericum	Sciatica. Nerve pain. Pinched nerve. Herniated disk. Spinal cord injury. Spasms after an injury. Tailbone pain. Injuries, especially from falling or from a blow.	Shooting pain from injured spot. Tingling, prickling, burning, numbness. Paralytic weakness. Shuddering. Painfully sensitive spine. Pain in nape of neck. Cervical vertebrae very sensitive to touch. Lower back pain. Violent pain and inability to walk after injury to coccyx. Joints feel bruised.	*Better:* Lying face down. Bending head back. *Worse:* Shock. Exertion. Jarring. Light touch. Change of weather, fogs, cold, damp.	Darting pains in shoulders. Crawling sensations in hands and feet. Jerks, sharps pains in the limbs. Limbs feel detached. Headache. Dizziness.	Nervous depression, especially after an accident. Melancholy. Irritable. Weak memory. Feels lifted high in the air, or is anxious about falling from a great height. Appetite increases in morning and evening. Great thirst. Drowsy. Talks wildly in sleep, especially after 4 A.M. Limbs jerk and twitch while sleeping.

Remedy	Helpful for	Sensation	Modalities	Concomitants	Mentals & Generals
Kali carbonicum	Fibromyalgia. Sciatica. Lower back pain. Hip disease. Overexertion.	Sharp, cutting, stitching pain. Throbbing. Back feels as if broken. Stiffness and paralytic pain. Burning in spine. Lower back feels weak, back and legs give out. Pain in kidney region, buttocks, hip joints, thighs.	*Better:* Motion. Warm humid weather. Open air. Sitting with elbows on knees. *Worse:* Cold air in cold weather. Drafts. Early morning. Sudden or unguarded motion. Hunger.	Joints give way. Tearing pains in limbs. Pain from hip to knee. Soles of feet very sensitive, limbs jerk if feet are lightly touched. Violent "sick" headache. Oppression of breathing.	Peevish, irritable, quarrelsome, weepy. Hypersensitive to pain, noise, touch. Never wants to be left alone. Desire for sweets and acids. Drowsy after eating. Talks in sleep. Awakes between 1 A.M. and 4 A.M., cannot get to sleep again.

Remedy	Helpful for	Sensation	Modalities	Concomitants	Mentals & Generals
Lycopodium	Sciatica (right side). Bone degeneration.	Burning between shoulder blades, like hot coals. Lower back pain. Stiff back. Emaciation around neck. Bubbling sensations. Numbness. Tearing pains in shoulder and elbow joints. Twitching and jerking.	*Better:* Motion. Warm drinks. Cool air. From uncovering (especially the head). *Worse:* Between 4–8 P.M. Cold food or drink. Sitting erect.	Bones ache at night. Shakes head without apparent cause. Facial contortions. Hands and feet numb; limbs go to sleep. Right foot hot, left cold. Gout. Gassy. constipation or diarrhea.	Nervous excitement and prostration. Wants to be alone, but wants someone nearby if needed. Cranky on waking; may wake from hunger. Great hunger easily satisfied or arising soon after a large meal. Craves sweets, warm food and drink.

Remedy	Helpful for	Sensation	Modalities	Concomitants	Mentals & Generals
Nux vomica	Lower back pain. Overexertion.	Piercing, sticking, tearing, burning, stinging pains. Twitching or spasms. Nerve pain through neck and shoulders. Sudden loss of power in arms and legs in morning. Lower back pain is aggravated by turning over in bed, the person may sit up in order to turn over without pain.	*Better:* Rest. In the evening. Wet weather. After a bowel movement. With heat. *Worse:* Much worse in the morning, especially 3 to 4 A.M. Lying down, must get up and walk. Mental exertion. Cold, especially cold dry air. Eating, especially overeating. Stimulants. Anger.	Arms and hands go to sleep. Legs go numb, knees crack while walking. Headache, nausea. Very sensitive to cold, the slightest draft or coolness aggravates symptoms. Perspires freely.	Driven, given to excesses (overeats, substance abuse, esp. stimulants and alcohol). Impatient, irritable, argumentative, oversensitive, touchy. Difficulty sleeping due to overactive mind or sensitivity to slight noises. Cannot sleep after 3 A.M., is awake until morning, then may doze.

Remedy	Helpful for	Sensation	Modalities	Concomitants	Mentals & Generals
Phosphorus	Inflammation. Degenerative diseases. Spinal cord and nerves. Osteomyelitis. Bone fragility. Sprains.	Burning in back. Pain as if broken, impedes all motion. Cramp, burning between shoulder blades. Weak spine. Stitching pain from coccyx to base of skull. Joints stiff with little pain, easily dislocated. Weak spells in joints.	*Better:* Cold food, air, and applications. Massage, rubbing. Sitting. Lying on right side. In the dark. *Worse:* Change of weather. Windy, stormy weather. Physical or mental exertion. Lying on left side, painful side, or back. Exertion.	Bleeding, hemorrhages. Totters while walking.	Excitable, impressionable. Fearful. Timid and irresolute. Wants sympathy. Craves cold, iced drinks. Craves chocolate. Ravenous hunger, hunger after eating, night eating. Catnaps. Sleepless before midnight. Sleepwalking. Vivid dreams.

Remedy	Helpful for	Sensation	Modalities	Concomitants	Mentals & Generals
Pulsatilla	Upper and lower back. Pain that extends to hips. Premenstrual and menstrual backache. Sciatica. Arthritis. Rheumatism. Joint pain. Overexertion.	Shooting pain in the nape and back, between shoulders. Pain in sacrum from sitting. Wandering, stitching pains. May be worse on the right side. Pressure, distension, throbbing. Constricting, congestive. Back feels bandaged.	*Better:* Breezes. Cold applications, air, food and drink. Walking or slow motion in open air. Erect posture. Lying with head high. *Worse:* Evening and at night. Heat. Pressure on painless side. Lying or sitting quiet. Wet weather.	Legs painful, feel heavy and weary (worse when limbs hang down). Pain in hip joint. Joints swollen and red. Pain in limbs shifts rapidly, alternates from side to side, may let up with a "snap." Menstrual or premenstrual headache.	Weepy, clinging. Moody and changeable. Craves company and sympathy; likes being fussed over. Feels better after being served "treat" foods. Imsomnia. Sleeps in the afternoon. Sleeps under blankets with a window open.

Remedy	Helpful for	Sensation	Modalities	Concomitants	Mentals & Generals
Rhus toxicodendron	Lower back pain, stiffness. Stiff neck. Joint pain. Rheumatic pain. Sciatica. Herniated disk. Sprain, strain. Overexertion.	Stiffness. Pain. Rheumatic pain (hot, painful swelling of joints). Tearing pain in tendons, ligaments. Bones ache. Sciatic pain, radiates from lower back and tears down the thighs. Pain between shoulders when swallowing.	*Better:* Continuous motion, walking, change of position, from stretching out limbs. Warm, dry weather. Rubbing affected area. Lying on something hard. *Worse:* Cold, wet, rainy weather. During and after sleep, sitting, or resting. At night.	Tingling or loss of sensation in feet or fingertips. Numbness, paralysis. Trembling after exertion. Itching, skin or scalp. Headache in base of skull, or one that begins in the forehead and creeps back.	Sad, listless, irritable. No appetite. Craves milk and cold drinks. Drowsy after eating. Apprehensive at night. Restless, cannot remain in bed. Sleepless before midnight. Frequent violent yawning. Heavy stuporous sleep. Wakes tired, stiff, sore.

Remedy	Helpful for	Sensation	Modalities	Concomitants	Mentals & Generals
Sepia	Lower back pain. Spasms. Rheumatism. Injury. Overexertion. Premenstrual and menstrual backache. Sciatica.	Weak, empty, hollow feeling in lower back. Aching in lower back. Icy coldness between shoulder blades or in lower back. Icy coldness between shoulder blades. Sudden pain, as if struck with a hammer. A "bearing down" pain in the lower back which may hinder breathing.	*Better:* Vigorous motion, exercise, dancing. With legs crossed. Pressing back against something hard. Warmth. Cold drinks, cold bathing. Open air. *Worse:* Cold air, snowy air, dampness, before thunderstorms.	Sudden prostration. Muscles jerk. Burning sensations in different parts of the body. Feels cold, even in a warm room. Stiffness. Restless limbs, twitching and jerking night and day. Coldness in legs.	Angry, sensitive, irritable, sulky. Averse to company or sympathy, yet dreads being alone. Sudden cravings and sudden satiety. Everything tastes too salty. Desires chocolate and acids; acids aggravate. Wakes frequently as if having been called.

Remedy	Helpful for	Sensation	Modalities	Concomitants	Mentals & Generals
Silica	Degenerative disease. Bone spurs. Strain, overexertion. Hip or joint disease. Inflammation. Injury. Sciatica. Arthritis. Rheumatism.	Pain runs up the back, toward the head. Stiff neck with headache. Burning. Spinal irritation. Weakness, sensitive to drafts on back.	*Better*: Any warmth. Humid weather. *Worse*: Change of weather. Cold air, drafts, damp. Physical or mental exertion, excitement. Touch. Pressure. Riding in car. After eating.	Limbs weak, cramping, feel paralyzed. Hands tremble when trying to do something. Feet icy cold and sweaty. Stitches in chest through the back. Painless throbbing in sternum. Headache while fasting.	Obsessed with fixed ideas. Fainthearted, anxious. Cries easily. Sensitive to cold, overdresses for warmth. Lack of appetite, excessive thirst. Restless sleep with nightmares and frequent starting. Talks in sleep, may sleepwalk.

Remedy	Helpful for	Sensation	Modalities	Concomitants	Mentals & Generals
Sulphur	Upper back pain: neck and shoulders. Lower back pain. Arthritis. Ankylosing spondylitis. Rheumatism. Sciatica.	As if vertebrae glided over one other. Drawing pain between shoulders. Stiffness, especially neck. Lower back pain extends to stomach. Joints stiff and swollen. Inertia and feebleness of tone. Unsteady gait. Walks stoop-shouldered, can straighten up only after moving.	*Better:* Dry, warm weather. Warm room and applications. Hot drinks. Lying on right side. *Worse:* Warmth of bed. Washing or bathing. Periodically, at noon and midnight. Periodic, every 7 days. Standing. Stooping, jarring, motion.	Itching, worse with heat. Top of head feels hot. Burning in palms of hands and soles of feet. Knees and ankles stiff. Hands trembling, sweaty. Migraine or migraine-like headache. Marked congestion. Red, engorged face.	Childish peevish in adults. Selfish, no regard for others. Irritable, depressed, thin and weak. Feels dull and stupid. Weak, faint, and hungry at 11 A.M. Desires sweets or salt; eating them may provoke nausea or vomiting. Catnaps, rather than sleeping. Wakes at the slightest noise.

Remedy	Helpful for	Sensation	Modalities	Concomitants	Mentals & Generals
Zinc	Spinal disorders. Neuralgia. Rheumatism.	Pain in small of back. Cannot bear to have back touched. Tension and stinging between shoulders. Tearing in shoulder blades. Spinal irritation. Dull aching in spine, worse sitting. Burning along spine.	*Better:* Hard pressure. Warm open air. Motion. While eating. Rubbing or scratching. *Worse:* Wine. Physical or mental exertion. Noise. Touch.	Stumbling, spastic gait. Totters while walking. Lameness, weakness. Trembling and twitching of various muscles. Feet in continuous motion, cannot keep still. Feet and legs feel as if bugs were crawling over them. Anemia. Eczema.	Lethargic. Weak memory. Defective vitality. Very sensitive to noise. Muddled, stupid, repeats everything said to her. Averse to work, to talk. Cries out during sleep; wakes frightened, staring. Feet in motion during sleep. Sleepwalking.

PART FOUR

ADDITIONAL INFORMATION

Glossary

Acute Related to episodic stress or fatigue. Transient pain that can be related to particular precipitating factors, e.g., cold or flu, an injury, periodic stress.

Aggravation A temporary increase in the severity of symptoms due to taking a remedy in too high a potency.

Chronic A condition that is constant or recurs frequently (at least twice a week) and that resists treatment. Chronic conditions are often, but not always, genetically based. *(Note*: Chronic conditions should not be subject to self-care, but rather evaluated and treated by an experienced homeopath.)

Concomitants Secondary symptoms. Concomitant symptoms help identify appropriate remedies.

Dilution and succussion *See*: Potentize.

Dose A unit of the remedy, usually 1–3 pellets or drops. (Also refers to the episode of taking the remedy.)

Generals A category of symptoms that includes eating and sleeping patterns, emotional states, and reactions to weather and interior environments.

Homeopathy A system for treating illness and injury with specially prepared substances, called remedies, that assist the body's efforts to heal itself. The remedies are taken singly, that is, one medicine at a time, in minute doses, and after careful assessment of a broad range of symptoms.

Homeopath Someone who practices homeopathy.

Law of cure A description of the progress of healing codified in the mid-1800s by Dr. Constantine Hering. His observations are that healing progresses from more vital organs and functions to less vital ones, that symptoms disappear in the reverse order from which they appeared, and resolve from top to bottom (that is, head to feet).

Like cures like The primary tenet of homeopathy; in classic texts this idea is often given in Latin as: *similia similibus curentur.* It means that substances that can create symptoms in a healthy person can, when prepared according to homeopathic principles, aid the body in curing those symptoms in someone who is ill.

Location The site of the symptoms, illness, or pain.

Materia Medica Latin for "materials of medicine." A catalog of remedies detailing their effects.

Mentals Symptoms that affect the mental plane, for example: forgetfulness, poor concentration, confusion, or faulty perceptions of one's surroundings.

Minimal dosing The smallest effective dose of remedy. This idea is one of the four basic precepts of homeopathic philosophy.

Modalities A description of what makes you or your symptoms better or worse. These may include warmth or coolness, pressure on the painful area, sitting up or lying down, fresh air, motion or stillness, weather, and eating or drinking in general or eating and drinking particular things.

Onset A description of how the illness began, for example: rapid, gradual, after an injury, after exposure to weather.

Particular(s) The specific set of symptoms you develop

in reaction to an illness. Some of these are specific to the illness, for example, a cough or a stuffy nose with a cold. Others are specific to the way you react to the illness; for example, you may wish to be left completely alone until you feel better and be irritable if disturbed, or you may have changes in your appetite or sleep patterns. The totality of your symptoms is matched against the remedy pictures to identify an appropriate remedy.

Peculiar(s) Symptoms that seem contradictory; for example, you may have chills but crave cold drinks, or you may have a frequent, urgent desire to urinate, but urinating is painful and scanty. In homeopathy, these unexpected combinations are often the most significant factors for determining an appropriate remedy.

Potentize Repeated dilution and succussion according to established homeopathic formulas to remove material components and isolate and activate the healing energy or vital force.

Provings An early form of clinical trials in which 100 healthy people were given a remedy and their reactions (symptoms elicited) were recorded. These records provided the source material for the various Materia Medica available.

Remedy A homeopathically prepared substance used to relieve illness. Remedies are available as pellets (a milk sugar base), as liquids, or as creams and gels.

Remedy picture The array of symptoms elicited in healthy people during a proving. These symptoms are cataloged in a Materia Medica and are the basis for recommending particular remedies for particular illnesses.

Repertorize The process of comparing a patient's symptoms against the illnesses cataloged in a repertory in order to recommend an effective remedy.

Repertory A reference book that details illnesses with their symptoms and suggests remedies that can alleviate them.

Sensation The specific way the symptoms feel, for example: bursting, crushing, prickly, shooting, stabbing.

Succussion A portion of the process of preparing homeopathic remedies in which the substance is agitated by tapping, shaking, or stirring. Succussion alternates with dilution and is credited with maintaining the efficacy of the original substance despite extensive dilution.

Symptoms The characteristic way that an illness manifests and the way in which you interact with the illness. Symptoms are the basis upon which remedies are recommended: The greater the consonance between the symptoms of the patient and the symptoms ascribed to the remedy, the more effective it will be.

Taking the case A diagnostic interview in which the homeopath asks a variety of questions to determine what your symptoms are in order to recommend an effective remedy. The interview may be short if the problem is an acute illness, such as a sore throat, or quite long (2–4 hours) if the illness is severe, complex, or chronic.

Totality of symptoms One of the basic precepts of homeopathy and the one that best reflects its holistic base. Before recommending a remedy, a homeopath will ask for a "body scan"—a head-to-toe review of how you are feeling—and also ask about your mental, emotional, and spiritual reactions to the illness. This information, the totality of symptoms, determines the selection of remedies.

Vital force The energy that distinguishes animate from inanimate beings. Also the active portion of a healing substance that is isolated by homeopathic dilution and succussion and instilled in the remedies.

Resources

Web site: Homeopathy Home Page
The homeopathy home page has searchable databases of practitioners, professional organizations, pharmacies, training programs, and veterinary institutions in the United States and abroad.

http://www.homeopathyhome.com/directory/usa/ organisations.html

Professional Associations, United States
These organizations maintain lists of qualified homeopaths and may provide referrals for a modest fee. Some offer classes and other information suitable for laypeople.

American Association of Naturopathic Physicians
2366 Eastlake Avenue, Suite 322
Seattle, WA 98102
phone: 206 328 8510

National Center for Homeopathy
801 North Fairfax, Suite 306
Alexandria, VA 22314
phone: 703 548 7790
fax: 703 548 7792
web site: www.homeopathic.org

North American Society of Homeopaths
122 East Pike St. Suite 1122
Seattle, WA 98122
phone: 206 720 7000

Professional Associations, United Kingdom
British Homeopathic Association
27A Devonshire Street
London W1N 1RJ
phone: 0171 935 2163

Council for Complementary & Alternative Medicine
179 Gloucester Place
London NW1 6DX
phone: 0171 724 9103
fax: 0171 724 5330

Society of Homeopaths
2 Artizan Road
Northampton NN1 4HU
phone: 01 604 621 400
fax: 01 604 622 622

Sources for remedies, United States
Some pharmacies and many health food stores carry
homeopathic remedies. The following companies distrib-
ute and/or manufacture homeopathic remedies. You may
buy individual remedies, combination remedies, or kits
that include several remedies for specific purposes, e.g.,

first aid, pediatric care. Some also sell instructional books
and tapes.

Boericke and Tafel, Inc.
2381 Circadian Way
Santa Rosa, CA 95407
phone: 707 571 8202
fax: 707 571 8237

Boiron USA
6 Campus Blvd. Bldg. A
Newtown Square, PA 19073
phone: 800 BOIRON-1 (800 264 7661)
web site: http://www.boiron.fr

Dolisos America, Inc.
3014 Rigel Avenue
Las Vegas, NV 89102
phone: 800 DOLISOS (800 365 4767)

Homeopathy Works
124 Fairfax Street
Berkeley Springs, WV 25411
phone: 304 258 2541
fax: 304 258 6335
web site: www.homeopathyworks.com

Luyties Pharacal Company
4200 Laclede Avenue
St. Louis, MO 63108
phone: 314 533 9600

Standard Homeopathic Company
P.O. Box 61067
204-210 West 131st Street
Los Angeles, CA 90061
phone: 800 624 9659

Sources for Remedies, United Kingdom

Ainsworths
36 Cavendish Street
London W1M 7LH
phone: 0171 935 5330
fax: 0171 486 4313

Galen Homoeopathics
Lewell Mill
West Stafford
Dorchester
Dorset DT2 8AN
phone: 01 305 263 996

Helios Homoeopathic Pharmacy
97 Camden Road
Tunbridge Wells
Kent TN1 2QR
phone: 01 892 536 393
fax: 01 892 546 850

Weleda (UK) Ltd.
Heanor Road
Ilkeston
Derbyshire DE7 8DR
phone: 01 602 309 319
fax: 01 602 440 349

Bibliography

Homeopathy
Organon of Medicine, 6th edition
by Samuel Hahnemann
translated by William Boericke, M.D.
B. Jain Publishers (P) Ltd., 1990

Pocket Manual of Homoeopathic Materia Medica
by William Boericke, M.D.
B. Jain Publishers Pvt. Ltd., 1990

*Lotus Materia Medica, Homeopathic and Spagyric Medi-
    cines*
by Robin Murphy, N.D.
Lotus Star Academy, 1995

Repertory of the Homoeopathic Materia Medica
by J. T. Kent
B. Jain Publishers Pvt. Ltd., 1989

Homeopathic Medical Repertory, A Modern Alphabetical Repertory
by Robin Murphy, N.D.
Hahnemann Academy of North America, 1993

Everybody's Guide to Homeopathic Remedies
by Stephen Cummings and Dana Ullman
Tarcher/St. Martin's Press, 1984

Homeopathic Remedies for Health Professionals and Lay People
by Dale Buegel, Blair Lewis, and Dennis Chernin
Himalayan Publishers 1978, 1991

How to Use Homeopathy
by Dr. Christopher Hammond
Element, 1991

The Science of Homeopathy
by George Vithoulkas
Grove Press, 1980

Backache
No More Aching Back, Dr. Root's Fifteen-Minute-A-Day Program for a Healthy Back
by Leon Root, M.D.
Signet, 1991

Healing Back Pain, The Mind-Body Connection
by John E. Sarno, M.D.
Warner Books, 1991

Relief From Chronic Backache
by Edmund Blair Bolles
Dell Medical Library, 1990

Back Pain, What Works!
by Joseph Kandel, M.D. and David B. Sudderth, M.D.
Prima Publishing, 1996

Your Aching Back, A Doctor's Guide to Relief
Augustus A. White III, M.D.
Fireside Simon & Schuster, 1990

New Perspectives in Health Care
from Kensington Books

__Cancer Cure $12.00US/$15.00CAN
The Complete Guide to Finding and Getting the Best Care There is
by Gary L. Schine with Ellen Berlinsky, Ph.D.   0-8217-024-5
Diagnosed with incurable cancer, author Gary L. Schine found the
treatment that led him back to full recovery and perfect health. Now,
in this inspiring and invaluable guide, he shows you how to take
charge of your illness, your treatment, and your recovery. Includes
a complete glossary of terms and a comprehensive resource guide.

__Health and Fitness in Plain English $14.00US/$19.00CAN
by Jolie Bookspan, Ph.D.   1-57566-288-4
If you care about keeping fit, you've been bombarded with exercise
and nutrition advice. This powerful guide cuts through the hype and
brings you the truth about top nutrition plans, permanent weight loss,
osteoporosis prevention, the biggest health food store rip-offs, and so
much more.

__The Brain Wellness Plan $14.00US/$19.00CAN
by Dr. Jay Lombard and Carl Germano, RD, CNS 1-57566-293-0
Now, a leading neurologist and renowned nutritional scientist bring
you the latest developments in brain research, as well as a comprehensive plan for building brain health. In fascinating, easy-to-under-
stand detail, this innovative bestseller guides readers through proven
medical, hormonal, and nutritional therapies that will help prevent
and treat disease.
